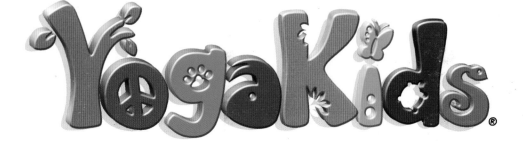

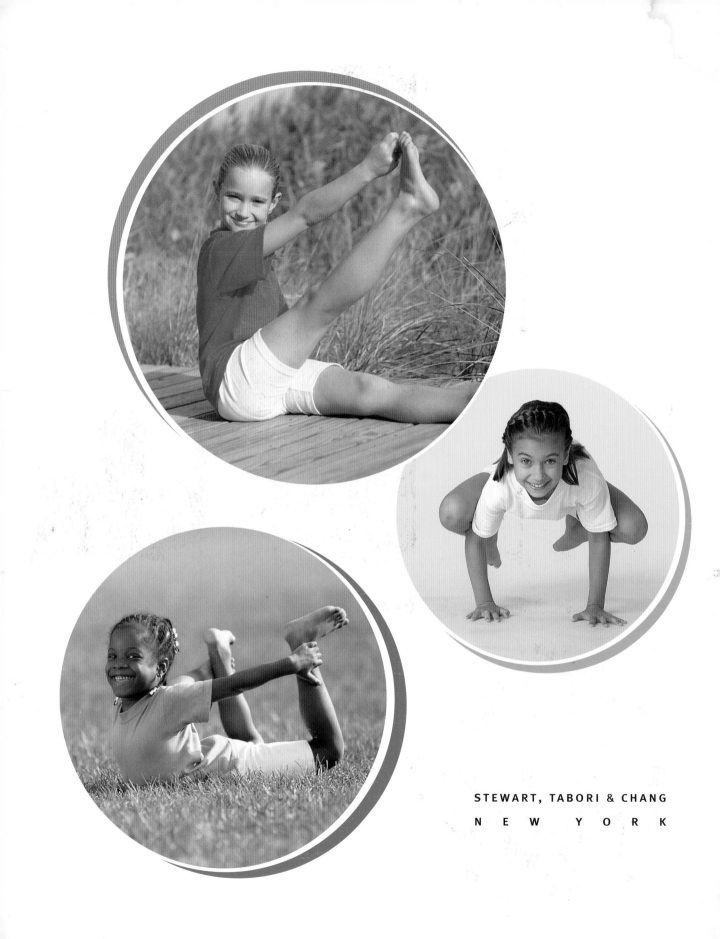

STEWART, TABORI & CHANG
N E W   Y O R K

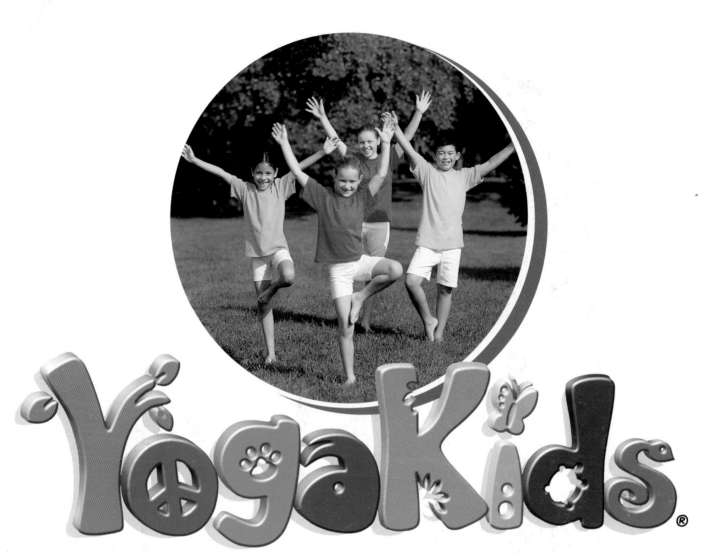

YogaKids

Educating the Whole Child through Yoga

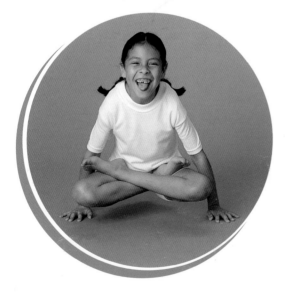

Marsha Wenig

Photographs by

Susan Andrews

Published in 2003 by Stewart, Tabori & Chang
A Company of La Martinière Groupe
115 West 18th Street
New York, NY 10011

Export sales to all countries except Canada, France and French-speaking Switzerland:
Thames & Hudson
181A High Holborn Ltd.
London WC1V 7QX
England

Canadian Distribution:
Canadian Manda Group
One Atlantic Avenue, Suite 105
Toronto, Ontario M6K 3E7
Canada

Library of Congress Cataloging-in-Publication Data

Marsha, Wenig
    YogaKids®: the whole-child program of learning through yoga/
By Marsha Wenig
    p. cm.
    ISBN 1-58479-292-2
1. Yoga, Hatha, for children. 2. Exercise for children. I. Title.

RA781.8.W465 2003
613.7'046'083—dc21   2003042448

Designed by Susi Oberhelman

Illustrations on p. 104-105 by Laurel Izard

YogaKids® is a registered trademark of Dancing Feet Yoga Center, Inc.

The exercises in this book are gentle and safe provided the instructions are followed carefully. However, the publishers and authors disclaim all liability in connection with the use of the information in individual cases. If you have any doubts as to the suitability of the exercises, consult a doctor.

PRINTED IN CHINA

10 9 8 7 6 5 4 3 2 1

FIRST PRINTING

This book is dedicated to children everywhere: Learning yoga at a young age will bring peace and light to us all.

In loving memory of my parents, Ruthie and Eric Loeb.

Namaste to my magnificent family: Don, Dakota, and Kiva. I love you.

Contents

Introduction

Swami Satchidananda, one of the most famous yogis of our time, was once asked in an interview, "Are you a Hindu?"

"No," he replied. "I'm an undo."

Over the past twenty years, two things have transformed me: yoga and motherhood. Both forced me to come undone, and in time, to come back together. The word *yoga* means, "to yoke." Teaching yoga to children has inspired me to slow down, has demanded that I practice what I preach, and continually allows me to educate in ways that encourage a peaceful mind, a healthy body, and a creative spirit. By bringing my two deepest passions together in a labor of love, I have been able to serve myself, my family, and my community.

YogaKids® teaches children to "bunny breathe" in order to boost energy when they're tired, to release their anger with explosion sounds in Volcano, and to focus before tests with "Take 5" breaths. When they practice the Warrior series with affirmations, their bodies grow stronger, and their confidence and self-esteem are enhanced. I love knowing that, at five years old, they're learning life skills I didn't have until my life nearly fell apart.

Back in the 1970s and '80s, I was a heavy smoker, a stressed-out professional woman whose past careers had included TV news producer, public relations VP, film music coordinator, and road manager for the singing group The Manhattan Transfer. Both of my parents passed on in a short span of time. My grief was great, and yoga became my solace.

For someone with a tense lifestyle and an overactive mind, yoga was the perfect antidote. Physically, it made me feel good. Mentally and emotionally, it steadied my nerves and helped me to relax. In a short time, I felt a new ease in my body.

I quit smoking, began teaching creative writing to children in the L.A. public schools, and met Don, my yoga instructor, who became my husband. The frazzled, nicotine-addicted woman I'd been years earlier became a distant memory. Don and I moved to the Midwest with our three-month-old daughter Dakota and opened the Dancing Feet Yoga and Retreat Center in Michigan City, Indiana.

While L.A. had a yoga studio on every other corner, Michigan City had misinformation and confusion about the practice. Our aim was to educate people about yoga, and their curiosity spurred our fledgling business.

Meanwhile, I was a "yoga mom," learning how to be a mother and practicing my craft every day to help me stay present, peaceful, and healthy. Dakota had been doing yoga with me since before she was born, in utero, and now I enjoyed her willingness to "play yoga." I wanted to branch out, share yoga with her and her friends. When her Montessori preschool accepted my offer to teach, I felt confident. After all, I'd been teaching yoga to adults for several years, and studying Iyengar yoga for almost a decade.

I was in for a surprise. Two classes later, my frustration nearly overcame me. Teaching children was nothing like teaching adults. I knew what wasn't working, yet I didn't know how to fix it.

Unlike adults, children didn't wait for my instructions, nor were they interested in explanations. They just jumped right in and did the poses *with* me. They had absolutely no interest in holding poses, or in trying harder or trying again. They wanted to play and have fun. Children live in the moment; those moments move fast, and the questions come even faster. Why is Dog pose Dog pose when it doesn't look like a dog? Dogs bark, nip heels, and lift their legs to pee; they don't look like little pup tents!

It was time to undo what I had learned.

I got off the mat and experimented. Dakota walked me around by my shirt collar in Down Dog while I barked and growled. We rolled around like puppies. She kissed me with licks. We hissed like snakes in *bhujangasana,* the Cobra pose, and I slithered out of my old skin. After my training from the children, yoga would never be the same. The kids began to call me Mrs. Yoga, and they became my beloved Yoga Kids.

Once I began to tune in to how they wanted me to teach them, we created amazing classes together. I continually modified traditional poses to make these age-old techniques child-friendly and fun. We played games, read books, learned anatomy, counted, sang songs, and put stuffed animals on our bellies as breathing buddies.

Yoga became the springboard to creativity and exploration. We did yoga *with* nature, and observed animal behavior. We played percussion instruments as we walked in kooky and rhythmic ways. We wove stories with both our bodies and minds. With this interdisciplinary approach, the classes were exciting, expressive, and alive. The children were hungry for movement through space; though they loved having their own mats, they didn't want to be confined to them.

If I had quieted the children and forced them to learn in a rigid, adult manner, they'd have quickly lost interest. But because we learned together, the children responded, and the YogaKids program blossomed.

Often when I leave a school, the children say, "I wish every day was a yoga day." Now it can be! This book is an introduction and guide to the YogaKids program, something you and your child can experience together in your home.

"Peace begins with me" is one of the affirmations the children say in YogaKids classes. This phrase helps them recognize they have the power to change the world, both internally and externally.

In your hands is the power to help your child develop a strong body, gain respect and love for herself, and discover a place of stillness and peace. YogaKids is a stepping stone on the journey. It brings that marvelous inner light that all children have to the surface. Watch them shine!

Namaste,
MARSHA WENIG

Foundations of YogaKids®

At its most fundamental, the YogaKids® program is about learning. Children are insatiably curious, and that's a wonderful thing. In the early days of the program—when YogaKids was just my daughter's preschool class and me—I faced dozens of children who'd never heard of yoga. Their spontaneity and constant questions both exasperated and inspired me, but I knew we could learn so much together. I was committed to teaching them yoga in ways that worked on all levels, from the physical to the subtle.

I wanted to engage their brains and hearts as well as their minds and bodies. In addition to the movement, we talked about animals, feelings, death—whatever came to their minds. I longed to use the practice of yoga to stimulate their capacity to learn and educate them completely.

People always say children are like sponges, and that's true, but each is a *different* kind of sponge. Children absorb and process information through moving, seeing, listening, touching, and even singing. Using all of these, we help develop every aspect of a child's mind, body, and spirit. No two children learn in exactly the same way.

Eight Intelligences

You may have heard of Howard Gardner's theory of multiple intelligences, developed in 1983 and described in his first book, *Frames of Mind*. Gardner named the seven intelligences all people exhibit: verbal/linguistic, logical/mathematical, visual/spatial, musical/rhythmic, body/kinesthetic, interpersonal, and intrapersonal. The more ways information can be processed, the more likely it will be stored in a variety of networks, and the more accessible it will be. It's like cross-referencing your mind: no matter which route you take to retrieve the information, you'll be able to get to it.

In the mid-1990s Gardner added "naturalist" to his list of intelligences, bringing the current count to eight: eight ways in which we understand the world, and eight ways that children learn.

Here's a quick look at the types of intelligences.

Verbal/linguistic intelligence is the ability to read, write, and communicate with words. Children who love rhyming, writing, talking, jokes, and storytelling are showing their linguistic ability.

Logical/mathematical intelligence is the ability to reason and calculate. Kids who love counting, math, problem solving, logic games, and baseball statistics show strength in logical/mathematical intelligence.

(These two kinds of intelligence are typically the most valued in our mainstream education system.)

Visual/spatial intelligence refers to the ability to draw, sculpt, paint, build, or navigate. These children love coloring, building blocks, jigsaw puzzles, sailing, and chess.

Body/kinesthetic intelligence processes information through touch, movement, dramatics, and, of course, yoga. These kids love sports, dancing, and any kind of movement system.

Musical/rhythmic intelligence involves recognizing patterns and rhythms, playing instruments, singing, rapping, and chanting. Most children learn the alphabet through this intelligence. Music and rhythm are powerful hooks to memory.

Interpersonal intelligence includes the skills of communicating, relating, sharing, and cooperating. These kids love working in groups and playing with other kids, and are often quite charming and personable.

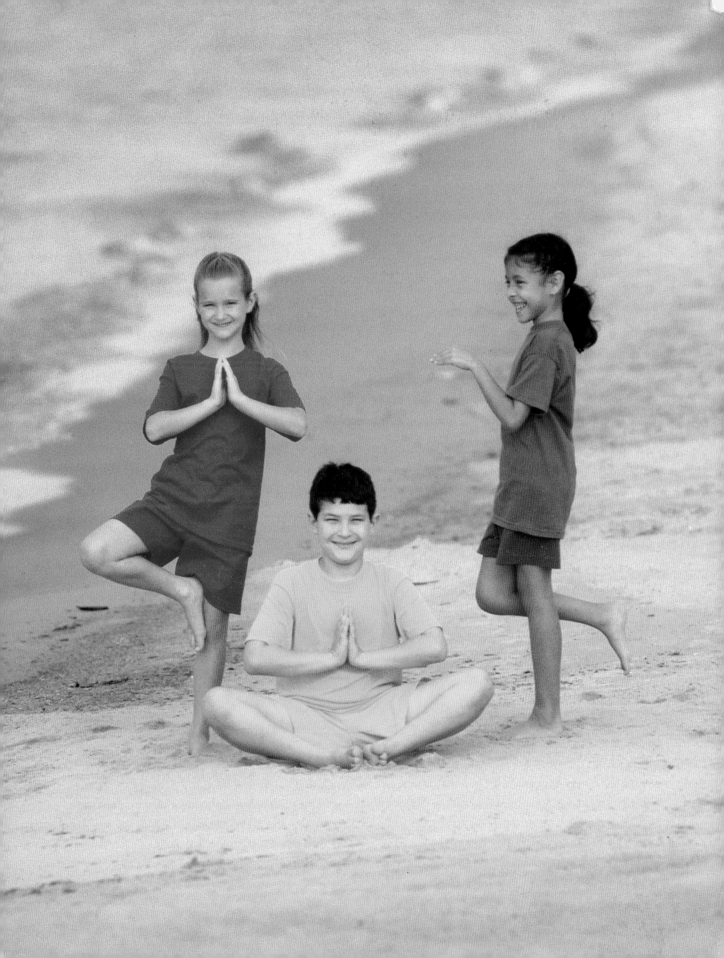

Intrapersonal intelligence is the introspective intelligence. These children generally develop insight, intuition, and self-reflection. They enjoy writing in journals, reading, spirituality, and philosophy.

Naturalist intelligence involves an awareness and interest in nature and their personal environment. These children love the outdoors, nature walks, taking care of plants and animals, watching nature shows, and reading stories about animals.

The Elements of YogaKids®

Gardner's theory, used with yoga as the medium of learning, led to the concept of the "elements" of YogaKids. They're designed to stimulate and teach a multitude of ways to perceive and access information. Together, the elements create a matrix for learning.

Poses as Pathways launches this whole-mind, brain-body, education system. The body moves into the poses, and the brain creates new neural pathways and increases its learning potential. A pose may help to teach math, ecology, anatomy, music, and more. The poses are the stepping stones to all of the other elements, which create even more avenues to learning.

Body Benefit describes how each pose benefits the physical body. Every pose has numerous physical benefits. Kids love learning how their bodies work, and they'll know they can use a particular pose, like 360-Degree Owl, for example, if their neck feels tight, or practice Mountain to help improve their posture.

Bridge of Diamonds combines the intrapersonal (communion with ourselves) and the interpersonal (the sense of community with others). As I tell the children, each one of us is a shining diamond: unique, multifaceted, and brilliant in our own way. Each of the poses creates a "bridge" that connects your child to the world—to nature, to you, and to his own body, mind, and spirit, too.

Brain Balance stimulates the communication of the body's systems: respiratory, nervous, and endocrine. With a combination of yoga movements and breathing techniques, the glands, hormones, and hemispheres of the brain are balanced. For example, in Eyes Around the Clock, the circular movement of the eyes engages the brain's superhighway (corpus callosum) to maximize the potential of the whole brain. This element was inspired by the work of Dr. Paul Dennison and his Brain Gym® program.

Ecological Echoes highlights our connection to the earth. We use yoga's animal and nature poses to share facts and environmental tips and reinforce the concept of interdependence. In Snake, for instance, children learn that snakes don't have ears, but they "hear" through the earth as they slither.

Math Medley uses mathematical concepts to highlight patterns, sequences, numerical awareness, counting, and rhythm while practicing poses. In Om a Little Teapot (Triangle), we describe three types of triangles.

Musical Musings develops an awareness and appreciation for sound and rhythm. Songs and simple percussive instruments, added to the movement, sharpen hearing, musical, and listening skills. For example, in Pedal Laughing, we move the body in rhythm with laughter and learn different music terms; *piano*, or quietly; *forte*, or loudly; and *adagio*, or slowly.

We All Win uses games and activities to promote cooperation and "win-win" thinking. Each child is recognized as an equal part of the whole. In Row Your Boat, we support each other in helping to maintain our balance.

Awesome Anatomy teaches bones, muscles and basic anatomical concepts to develop health and body awareness. In Peanut Butter and Jelly, we "smear" peanut butter all over our body parts, identifying each one as we do it. Smaller children use common names for parts of the body, while older children can learn the scientific names.

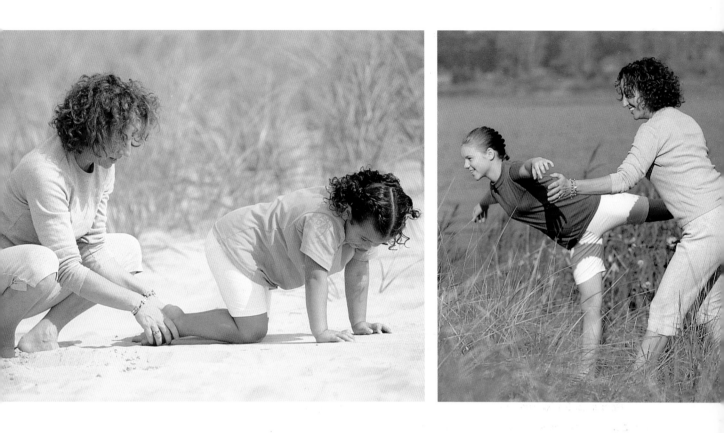

Reading Comes Alive (with Yoga) uses yoga to enhance reading skills. We do yoga poses that follow along with a story, and help children retain story sequence and characters. With Jules Pfeiffer's *Bark George,* for example, we practice Moo and Meow, Down Diggety Doggy Down, and other poses. (See page 118.)

Laughing Language encourages children to play with words and have fun with language. When presented in the context of play, they're more likely to become creative and free in their expression. ABC poses, for instance, are great ways to teach sounds, alliteration, and rhyming, as in R Is for Roar, in which your child will learn how to speak lion-ese!

Visual Vignettes explores thematic ways to use clay, paint, crayons, and craft ideas to develop visual skills and reinforce poses and other elements. In Ankle-Heel-Toe Walking, for example, we trace each other's feet and learn all of their parts (this involves Awesome Anatomy, as well).

Affirmations use positive messages that encourage and reinforce peacefulness, confidence, joy, honesty, and compassion in our children. In the Warrior series, strength of the body and determination is reaffirmed with verbalizations such as "I am strong."

Quiet Quests highlights and expands on the introspective aspects of yoga: meditation, concentration, focus, breathing, and relaxation. Kids learn to use yoga to calm, rest, and center themselves. Doing Swim Ducky Swim before bed, for instance, is very restful and calming for children. Like math and reading, Quiet Quest skills will serve them well all their lives.

All of the elements integrate exercise and physical learning with intellectual growth, music, the arts, and other creative and life-enhancing skills. If it seems a bit overwhelming, don't worry. Have fun exploring and let your creativity flow. As soon as you begin to do the program, you and your child will be exercising, educating, and enjoying yoga together in no time.

How to Use this Book

This book is a tool you and your child can use together. It's *not* a training manual for YogaKids® instructors (aka Certified YogaKids Facilitators, or CYKFs). Our facilitators have years of experience with yoga, intensive training with the YogaKids methodology and child development, and experience working with large groups of children in class settings. But you really need not have any experience with yoga to use this version of the program successfully at home. You know your child's needs and abilities, and the book will explain the rest.

You can do some or all of the poses. You can also decide where to do the poses, and which of the elements you and your child will do. I have included a number of sequences, or routines, of yoga poses, designed to meet you and your child's particular goals of the moment—whether you have fifty minutes to practice yoga, or five.

Before digging into the poses, though, you and your child may choose a few extra items to work with.

Good to Have

- **Sticky mats.** Most yoga classes use sticky mats, which offer a nonslip surface for better traction in standing and balancing poses. Although it's not essential, I feel it's important, and children enjoy having their own space and boundaries. A towel, small blanket, or rug will also do.

- **A basket or container filled with supplies for the elements.** These supplies might include crayons, markers, paints, paper, scissors, writing utensils, a ruler, tape measure, and a drawing compass.

- **A basket filled with "focus friends" and "breathing buddies."** A rubber ducky, small stuffed animals, beanbag toys, or any special objects that your children choose will help them focus for poses that require relaxation or concentration.

- **Books and music.** You might also have some of your favorite "Reading Comes Alive" books on hand and a CD or tape player to play music. (See page 114–122 for recommendations.)

Fun to Have

- **Blankets.** You can use these to "tuck children in like an enchilada" or "wrap them up like Dracula" in Lemon Toes, the YogaKids variant of the Corpse pose. (See page 100.)

- **Herbal eye pillows.** These help children completely relax, draw inward, and lie still.

- **A small bottle of lotion and essential oils.** Most children (and probably you, too) love to have their feet rubbed at the end of their relaxation session. Keep a small bottle of lotion on hand, along with some of your favorite essential oils, like peppermint or lavender. Add a few drops to make your own blend.

- **Percussion instruments.** For certain poses like Ankle-Heel-Toe Walking, it's nice to have some rhythm sticks, hand drums, or simple percussion instruments to create Musical Musings.

- **Bare feet.** Yoga is practiced with your socks and shoes off. Wear nonrestrictive, comfortable clothing on the rest of your body.

Location

You can practice inside or out. Select a quiet, clean spot without too many distractions. Please practice with the television and radio off! Outside is wonderful, if the weather is pleasant. Children like familiarity, so try to designate one area as your special yoga place. Allow your child to leave all her equipment there, along with this book, so she can practice on her own.

Time

Select the best time for you and your child. I like doing yoga in the morning, because it's a great way to wake up. Yoga before bedtime is an excellent way to wind down, relax, and prepare for sweet dreams. Your child will have favorite poses; encourage him to practice these poses whenever he feels like it. I've included sequences for different times of the day. (See pages 18–19.)

Take little yoga breaks throughout the day. With time and practice, you and your child will naturally integrate different poses into your daily routines.

Practice for as long as it is enjoyable. Ten to thirty minutes is probably average.

Please do not practice after eating a large meal. On the other hand, practicing on an "empty" stomach isn't practical. Aim for two or three hours after a meal, even though with children that's usually not possible since hungry children make cranky children! Just do the best you can.

Feel Good About It!

We want children to know that physical and mental fitness is an enjoyable and essential process.

YogaKids might or might not create a yogi out of your child, but it allows you to bond and share time together with a wholesome activity that helps your child learn about his or her body, mind, environment, and creativity.

Using the elements, let the poses flow into reading, writing, drawing, art, and music. I feel completely confident that this book will give your family tools for health, fitness, relaxation, and education that will last a lifetime.

You know your child best, so go at his pace and encourage him, and you'll both have much more fun.

Sharing yoga with children helps them

- Feel loving and loved.

- Get in touch with themselves and learn to trust their instincts.

- Learn about their bodies.

- Acknowledge and nurture their special gifts and strengths.

- Experience fun, playfulness, and collaboration with others in the learning process.

- Open up to change, ask questions, and find their own answers.

- Uncover their innate sense of joy.

- Know that the quiet, still place within is there for them, through the changes, challenges, and confusion of growing up.

- Fill up with vibrant, vital energy. (In yoga, we call it *prana*.)

- Demystify yoga by having it served up in child-sized portions.

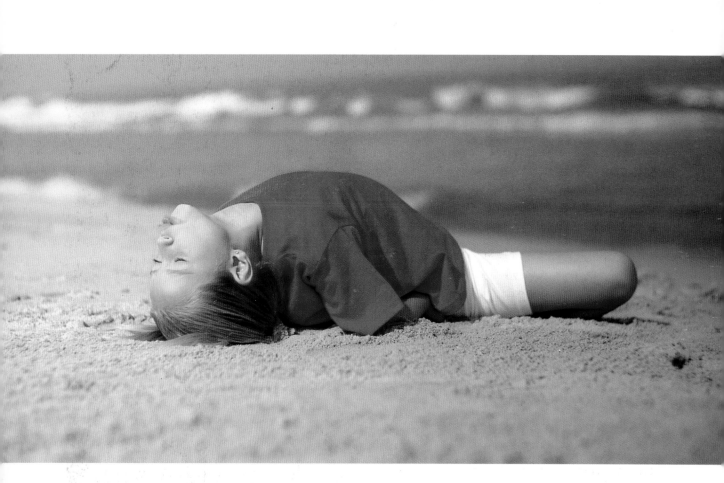

Find the routines you love and do those over and over, or do a different one every day. We know kids are very sensitive to adults' moods; if you're overcritical, they're anxious. And if you're relaxed, so are they! You might feel foolish at first, making dog noises and shaking like jelly, but once you start thinking like a kid and acting like a kid, you'll discover a world of fun you left behind. Many of our CYKFs are actually using YogaKids® techniques in their adult classes, and the response has been nothing short of wonderful: "It's freeing and liberating and so much more fun than regular yoga!"

If you've taken yoga before, you might be inclined to try to do the poses "perfectly" and make sure your child does the same. My only advice for this is: Don't. Save it for your adult yoga class. If your child's feet are slightly out of place, or if they're not epitomizing the perfect Warrior pose, that's okay. As long as you're

As with any exercise program, consult your doctor or health care practitioner before beginning. The poses in this book range from full-body movements and inversions to eye exercises and relaxation, so kids of any ages and abilities can achieve some semblance of the poses. For the more difficult poses, like the handstand, be there to spot your child.

Always try to achieve comfort in the asana. The word *asana* (pose or posture) really means "to take a comfortable seat." So do not force or strain, but practice gradually and gently. Never hold your breath. Keep your body and breath flowing in an even rhythm, and just do your personal best.

both having fun and learning together, you're achieving the goal of YogaKids. The intention is to build a lifelong foundation for yoga, so they will continue to practice forever. Over time and with repeated practice, their technique and form will continue to refine and improve.

Yoga with Children of Different Ages

Make yoga a special time for you and your child. Let go of expectations. Move out of your habitual way of being with other people. No ordering or judging—just fun! They'll get the poses on whatever level they can.

Ages 2–6: Kids this age love to role-play and pretend, so just let them be who they are. Their attention spans may seem short, but they're always paying attention and absorbing information on some level. They're learning even when they're not doing. And if a small child gets caught up in making snake noises and slithering across the floor instead of continuing with the poses, that's fine. Make the sound with her and talk about being unafraid of snakes. Children don't like holding poses, as adults do, but they do enjoy constant activity, so you just might have trouble keeping up with them.

Some poses may be too difficult for younger children. Use your best judgment of the child's ability, and let her move at her own pace.

Ages 7–11: These children will generally show marked improvement as they practice, but the key is not to correct them too much. Children this age are especially sensitive to criticism, and if they perceive themselves as not good at something now, they may never want to try it again. YogaKids is about developing a love for learning and yoga early on; encouragement is the best method I know to lead children to continue with yoga on their own. It makes all the difference in the world. In addition, encourage them to help the younger children; when they realize how much they really know, they'll feel empowered to continue their own studies.

Dos and Don'ts

- **DO** say "Good job" often.

- **DON'T** tell your child to calm down.

- **DO** use this book to help her learn to relax and to know when she needs to "chill."

- **DON'T** feel that you always have to be quiet when you practice.

- **DO** integrate the songs and sounds of YogaKids® with your poses.

- **DON'T** phrase assistance negatively: "That's the wrong way," or "Don't do that!"

- **DO** phrase assistance positively: "How about this way?" or "Let's do this!"

- **DON'T** try to make your child do the poses perfectly.

- **DO** have fun.

- **DON'T** dictate.

- **DO** guide.

- **DON'T** give a lot of instructions all at one time. Teach her step by step, one direction at a time.

- **DON'T** discourage him when he gets off track. Redirect him back to the practice in gentle ways.

The Basics of the Program

Awesome Anatomy

Experiential learning is the best teacher. So as you and your child practice the yoga poses, it's a perfect opportunity to begin naming and understanding some of the major bones, muscles, and organs of the body. Many of the pose pages present an Awesome Anatomy element. Please refer to the anatomy chart on page 104, which lists common and more scientific names. Refer to the reading on page 122 for other child-friendly anatomy books and tools.

Poses as Pathways to Learning

The Poses are divided into the following sixteen sections.

- **Peace & Quiet**. Breathe your way to harmony and serenity.
- **Senses**. Experience your eyes, ears, heart, and soul.
- **Brain Balance**. Brainpower happens when both sides work together.
- **Strength & Courage.** Poses to build confidence, self-esteem, and power.
- **Shake Like Jelly.** Shake, loosen, and flop.
- **Four-Legged Friends**. Poses with four limbs; three mammals and a reptile.
- **Connecting**. Poses that bond, share, and unite.
- **ABCs**. Body language—from tongue to toes.
- **Feathers**. Bird poses that promote balance, poise, and grace.
- **Wet**. Poses that swim, spout, bubble, and paddle.
- **Moving & Grooving**. Active poses to keep energy moving onward and upward.
- **Pattern & Rhythm**. Repetitive movements that flow.
- **Shape & Form**. Poses that bend, rock, and move.
- **Edible**. Poses good enough to eat.
- **Upside Down**. Poses that invert the body for a new point of view.
- **Completion**. Poses of rest, relaxation, and renewal.

Each section contains a handful of poses and can even be practiced as a mini-lesson or sequence on its own. Say the name of the section and the name of the pose with your child as you do it, so she'll remember how each pose fits into YogaKids®. For instance, if she remembers that Take 5 is a Peace & Quiet pose, then she knows she can do Take 5 when she wants to feel peaceful.

Breathing Fundamentals

The breath is so simple, really. It's literally under our noses, but we often forget to breathe. One of the main principles separating yoga from other forms of exercise is to maintain a constant awareness of your breath. The breath oxygenates the organs, muscles, and cells of the body, as well as soothing and calming the nervous system.

In the Peace & Quiet poses and throughout the book, you will be introduced to various breathing techniques to practice with your child. We want to make the children aware of the power of the breath, without boring them with too much detail. They can learn the process experientially and with the help of the YogaKids elements, of course.

Remember the Breathing Basics

- **Unless otherwise instructed, breathe in and out through the nose.**
- **An inhalation is breathing in. An exhalation is breathing out. We do not recommend breath retention for children.**
- **Generally, we expand or move on an inhalation and contract or surrender on an exhalation.**
- **Breathe slowly and deeply.**

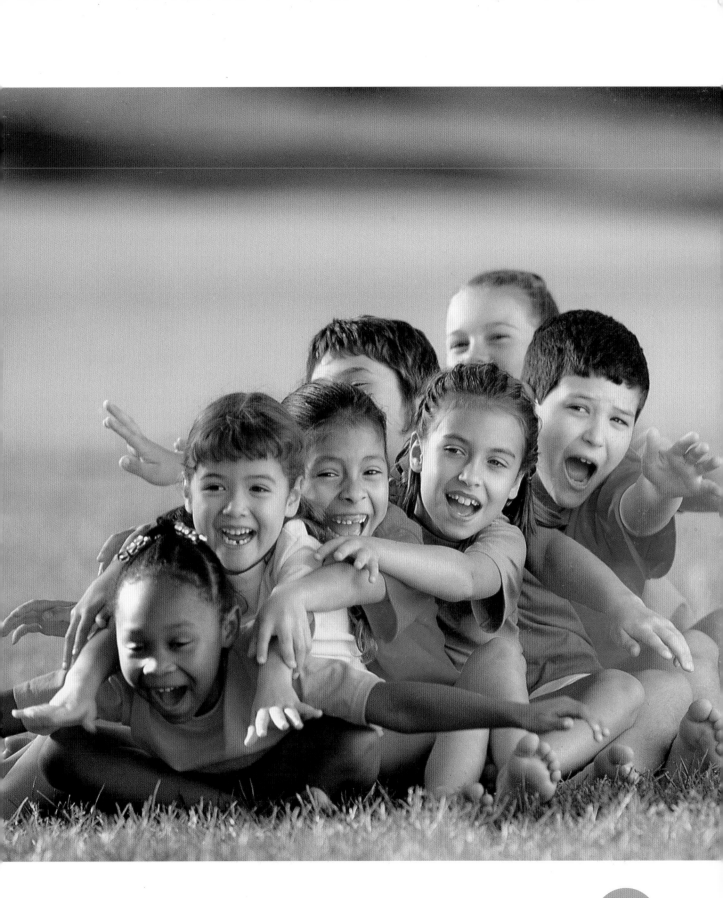

YogaKids® Sequences

Beginners

Peace Breath (25)
Bunny Breath (27)
Hot Air Balloon (29–31)
S Is for Snake (68)
R Is for Roar (67)
Butterfly (32)
Moo and Meow (38)
Mountain (49)
Jumpings (20)
Om a Little Teapot Triangle
  (88–89)
Warrior Series (54–55)
Reach for the Sun (86–87)
Volcano (50–53)
Stork (58–59)
Tree (56)
Twist and Blow (47)
Lemon Toes (100)
The Sound of Om (109)
Namaste song (113)

Advanced

Dragon Breath (28)
Pretzel (94)
Swinging Pretzel (94)
Talking Turtle (78–79)
Crow (61)
Down Diggety Doggy Down
  (40–41)
Spouting Dolphin (74)
Lizard (39)
Rocking Horse (90)
Dromedary Delight (42–43)
Wheel (91)
Handstand (98–99)
Birthday Candle Series (95–97)
Bubble Fish (80)
Twist and Blow (47)
Lemon Toes (100)

Waking Up

Hot Air Balloon (29–31)
Butterfly (32)
Moo and Meow (38)
Down Diggety Doggy Down
  (40–41)
Spouting Dolphin (74)
Reach for the Sun (86–87)
Tarzan's Thymus Tap (36)
Volcano (50–53)
Rocking Horse (90)
Dragon Breath (28)
Bunny Breath (27)

For 3-year-olds

Tarzan's Thymus Tap (36)
Bunny Breath (27)
Hot Air Balloon (29–31)
R Is for Roar (67)
Butterfly (32)
S Is for Snake (68)
Snake Charmer (69)
Rocking Horse (90)
Polar Bear (77)

Before Bed

Twist and Blow (47)
Take 5 (26)
Peace Breath (25)
Child's Pose (33)
Polar Bear (77)
Stork (58–59)
Lemon Toes (100)
Swim Ducky Swim (24)
Magical Cloud Carpet Ride (108)

Posture

Mountain (49)
Volcano (50–53)
Eagle (48)
Om a Little Teapot Triangle
  (88–89)
Warrior Series (54–55)
Tree (56)
Stork (58–59)
Moo and Meow (38)
Down Diggety Doggy Down
  (40–41)
Lizard (39)
Dromedary Delight (42–43)
Birthday Candle Series (95–97)
Butterfly (32)

Energize

Reach for the Sun (86–87)
Transformers Series (81–85)
Warrior Series (54–55)
Tarzan's Thymus Tap (36)
Dragon Breath (28)
Bow and Arrow (46)
Row Your Boat (76)

Calm

Peace Breath (25)
Child's Pose (33)
Extended Child's Pose (33)
Polar Bear (77)
Twist and Blow (47)
Swim Ducky Swim (24)
Lemon Toes (100)

Before a Test

Tarzan's Thymus Tap (36)
Eyes Around the Clock (34–35)
Bunny Breath (27)
Dragon Breath (28)
Bow and Arrow (46)
Mountain (49)
Eagle (48)
Ragdoll Ann and Ragdoll Andy (45)
Reach for the Sun (86–87)
Warrior Series (54–55)
Volcano (50–53)

Study Aids

R Is for Roar (67)
Bow and Arrow (46)
Moo and Meow (38)
360-Degree Owl (60)
Dromedary Delight (42–43)
Eagle (48)
Volcano (50–53)
Tarzan's Thymus Tap (36)
Warrior Series (54–55)

Crazy to Calm

Shake Like Jelly (45)
Untying the Knots (44)
Bug-Pickin' Chimp (71)
Ankle-Heel-Toe Walking (70)
Reach for the Sun (86–87)
Volcano (50–53)
Warrior Series (54–55)
Tree (56)
Stork (58–59)
Bunny Breath (27)
Peace Breath (25)
Child's Pose (33)
Polar Bear (77)
Lemon Toes (100)

In the Car

Bunny Breath (27)
Peace Breath (25)
Eyes Around the Clock (34–35)
Butterfly (32)
360-Degree Owl (head only) (60)
Electric Circle (62)
Lizard Tongue (39)
Lemon Toes (seated) (100)

Small Spaces

Butterfly (32)
360-Degree Owl (60)
Rocking Horse (90)
Child's Pose (33)
Polar Bear (77)

Forward and Back

All Fours (20)
Down Diggety Doggy Down
    (40–41)
Spouting Dolphin (74)
S Is for Snake (68)
Swan (81)
Child's Pose (33)
Polar Bear (77)
Seesaw Triangle (65)
Talking Turtle (78–79)
Row Your Boat (76)
Rock 'n' Roll (95)
Bridge (97)
Bow and Arrow (46)
Rocking Horse (90)
Dromedary Delight (42–43)
Peanut Butter & Jelly (92–93)
Extended Child's Pose (33)

Body Geometry

Transformers Series (81–85)
Om a Little Teapot (88–89)
Warrior Series (54–55)
Handstand (98–99)
Child's Pose (33)
Polar Bear (77)
Spouting Dolphin (74)
Rock 'n' Roll (95)
Birthday Candle Series (95–97)
Plough (96)
Bridge (97)
Wheel (91)
Twist and Blow (47)

Body Concert

Pedal Laughing (37)
Row Your Boat (76)
Rocking Horse (90)
Bug-Pickin' Chimp (71)
Down Diggety Doggy Down
    (40–41)
Spouting Dolphin (74)
Tarzan's Thymus Tap (36)
Ankle-Heel-Toe Walking (70)
Om a Little Teapot Triangle
    (88–89)

Just for Fun

Untying the Knots (44)
Shake Like Jelly (45)
Ragdoll Ann and Ragdoll Andy
    (45)
Bug-Pickin' Chimp (71)
Down Diggety Doggy Down
    (40–41)
Hot Air Balloon (29–31)
Pedal Laughing (37)

Base Poses

Certain postures work as starting positions for many of the poses in this book.

1. All Fours
From the Heel Sitting position (see photo 4), bring your hands, fingers outstretched, forward and set them down, with your wrists slightly in front of your shoulders. Your knees are under your hips, and your feet stretch straight back.

2. Pretzel Sitting
Instead of crossing your ankles under your knees, as in a regular cross-legged position, cross them and place them on top of your thighs, so they are above your knees.

3. L Sitting
Sit on the floor with your legs stretched straight out in front of you. Feet are flexed. Stretch your spine tall.

4. Heel Sitting
Bend your knees and sit down on your heels. Angle your toes toward each other and your heels away from each other. Place your hands wherever they are comfortable, or follow the instructions for the individual pose.

5. Mountain
Stand tall, with your feet together. Let your arms hang at your sides, your fingers stretch downward.

6. Open Mountain
Same as Mountain, only the feet are hip-width apart. (For further instructions, see page 49.)

7. Namaste
(See page 9 for example.) The Hindu greeting is pronounced "Nah-mah-stay." Place your hands and fingers together at the heart. The Namaste position can be taken seated or standing.

8. Jumpings
Stand in Mountain pose, bend your elbows out to the side, and place your fingertips, with palms facing downward, together at chest level. Take a breath and jump your feet apart. Stretch your arms outward at shoulder height. Take a breath and jump your feet back together.

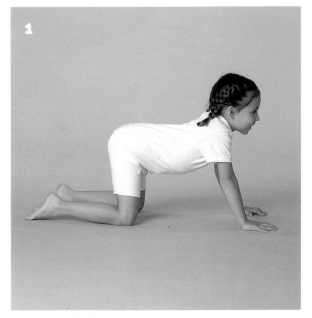

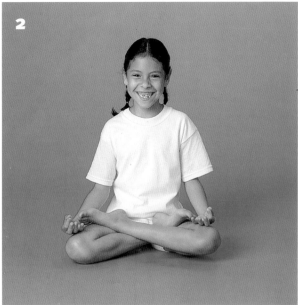

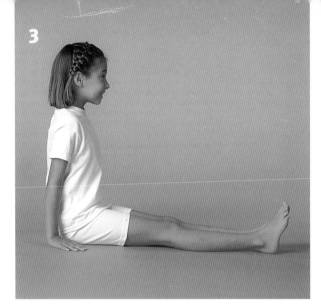

3

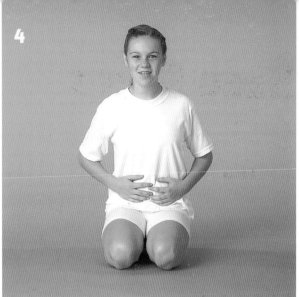

4

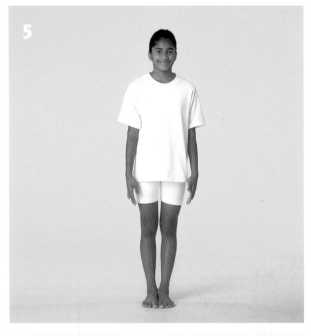

5

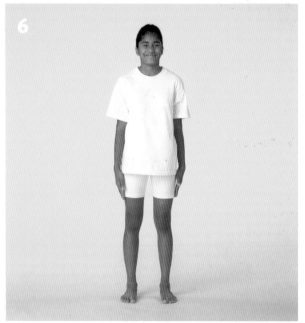

6

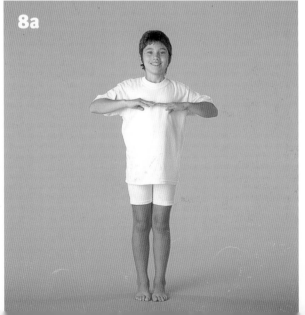

8a

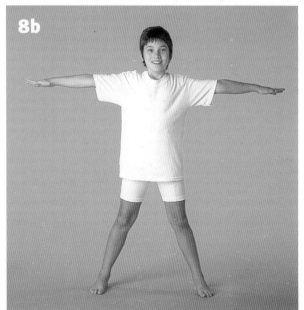

8b

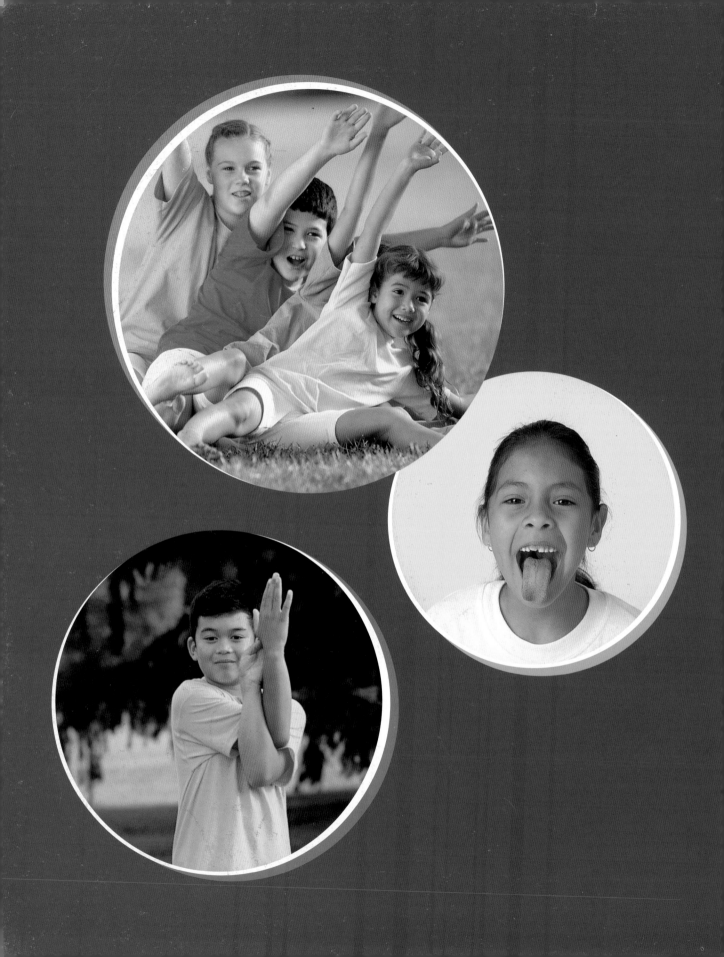

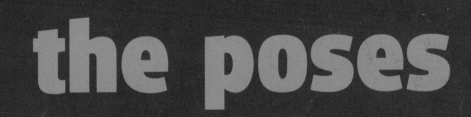

the poses

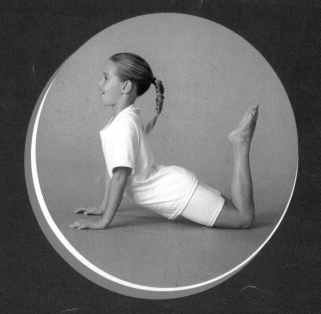

Swim Ducky Swim

Oxygen is brain food, so the more you practice this breath, the smarter you'll be! Your ducky will help you see that you're doing it right.

Lie down on your back. Place a rubber ducky on your belly. Breathe gently in (your belly button rises) and out (your belly button sinks down). As your belly rises and falls like the waves, your ducky surfs the waves as you inhale (breathe in) and floats as you exhale (breathe out). Give your ducky a slow and gentle ride with your breathing.

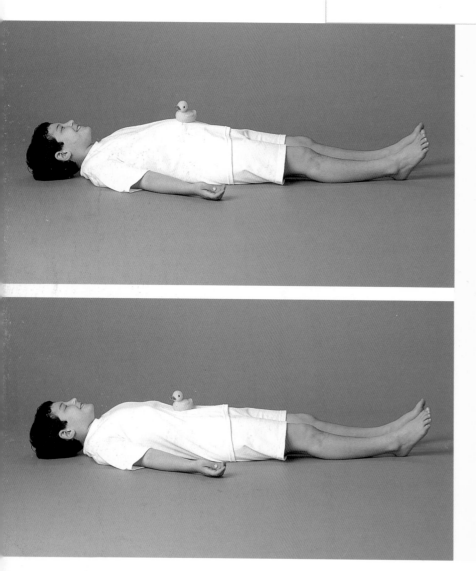

Elements

This technique helps children understand how to breathe completely using diaphragmatic, or belly, breathing.

The diaphragm is a muscle just below the lungs. It moves like an elevator—up and down. It goes down when you *inhale* (breathe in) and up when you *exhale* (breathe out), allowing your lungs to fill and empty completely.

Awesome Anatomy

Air comes into our bodies through our nose and mouth and travels down the trachea or windpipe, through the bronchial tubes, and into our lungs. Trace the air's path along your mouth and neck.

Quiet Quests

This is great at bedtime. Tell your child: Put a rubber ducky or your favorite stuffed animal on your belly. Use your breath to help your animal friend move in different ways. If you choose a bird, then your breath will help her fly. If it's a frog, your breath will help her leap.

peace & quiet

Peace Breath

Close your eyes. Relax your face muscles. Let your skin drape over your bones like a soft blanket. Breathe in. Breathe out, and whisper the word "peace." Do this 3 to 6 times. As you say the word, feel the peace inside you. Send peace to the animals, trees and plants. Send peace to your family. Send peace to countries in the world that are at war. Send peace to all the people you love.

Peace has many meanings. Love. Nonviolence. Compassion. Harmony. The peace breath is an easy way to feel peace. When you are peaceful, you will help everyone around you feel peaceful too.

Elements

Visual Vignettes
What does peace look like? Using one large sheet of paper, paint a picture of peace with your whole family or with a group of friends.

We All Win
This game of War and Peace strengthens your skills of tolerance and peace. One person is War. She makes mean, angry, and hateful comments to the other person, who is Peace. No matter what War says or does, Peace remains calm, by doing the Peace breath, and saying and sending peace to War. Then they switch roles.

Awesome Anatomy
Send peace to all parts of your body. When you have a tummy ache, send peace to your tummy. When you're angry or sad, send peace to your heart. When you hurt yourself, send peace to the hurt part.

Laughing Language
Learn the word for "peace" in different languages:

Arabic	*Salaam*
Cantonese	*Peng On*
Hebrew	*Shalom*
Hindi	*Shanti*
Russian	*Mir*
Spanish	*Paz*

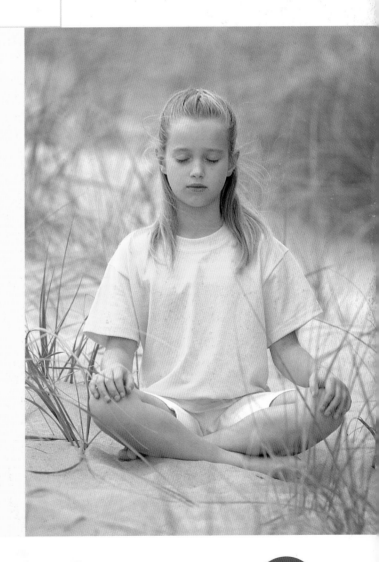

Take 5

"Take 5" means to take a break. Take 5 gives you a quick rest whenever you need it. Take 5 will also help you focus and concentrate.

Sit cross-legged. Lift one finger at a time as you breathe in through your nose and count in your mind: 1, 2, 3, 4, 5. (Or ask someone else to count out loud for you.) Pause for a second with your hand up. Slowly breathe out through your nose. Count backward—5, 4, 3, 2, 1—putting down one finger at a time for each number. Do "Take 5" 2 or 3 times.

Elements
This technique can be used anytime, anywhere, in any position to calm down and relax. Children love to remind their parents to "take 5" when they see them stressed or anxious. Over time, you'll just signal each other by holding up your hand in high-five or by humming the classic "Take 5" tune. You'll know what to do.

Math Medley
Increase your breath count by fives. Count to 10, then 15, then 20. The more you practice, the more your breath span will increase.

Quiet Quests
Begin and end your day with rounds of Take 5. Awaken with it. Fall asleep with it. Use it anytime to help calm and center yourself and your child.

Musical Musings
Play the classic jazz composition by Dave Brubeck, "Take 5" (see page 116). It's a catchy melody, and after a while you can just hum it as a signal to "chill" and take 5.

Bunny Breath

Get comfortable in a seated pose, such as L Sitting or Heel Sitting (page 20). Make your neck and back as long as you can, tuck in your chin slightly and let your lower jaw relax. Take 4 to 6 short, quick breaths in through your nose. Twitch your nose like a bunny. Then breathe out through your mouth with a long, smooth sigh. Repeat four times. Does your bunny feel energized?

Increase the number of inhalations and double the length of your exhalations as your breath power gets stronger.

Bunny Breath cleans the inside of your body like a washcloth and soap cleans the outside.

Elements

This technique is a quick pick-me-up. Children can use it to boost their energy and clear their minds.

All breathing poses are especially helpful for children with ADD and ADHD.

Quiet Quests

This breath calms and energizes at the same time. It gives you a feeling of relaxed alertness, which is an optimum state for learning.

Brain Balance

The rapid intakes of oxygen inherent in this technique provide the brain with essential fuel. With enough Bunny Breath, you may begin to feel your brain as it charges up.

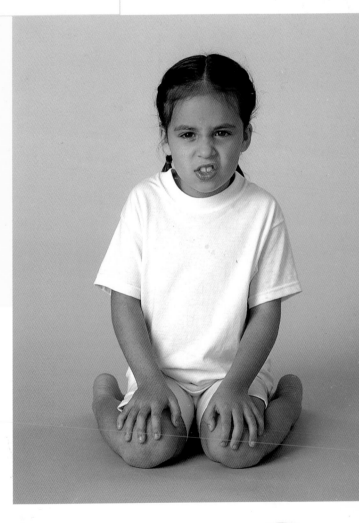

Dragon Breath

Dragons are said to breathe fire, and so can you when you do this pose.

Sit comfortably in any of the seated poses. Place your hands on your belly. Breathe out through your nose with a strong snort as you snap your belly back toward your spine. Focus on your breath as it goes out. A little bit of air will naturally sneak into your nose after each snort, so you don't need to think about inhaling, it will happen naturally. Do the Dragon Breath 3 to 6 times. Then breathe in and out normally. Add more rounds of Dragon Breaths as you feel comfortable. Your Dragon Breath will get stronger and longer with practice.

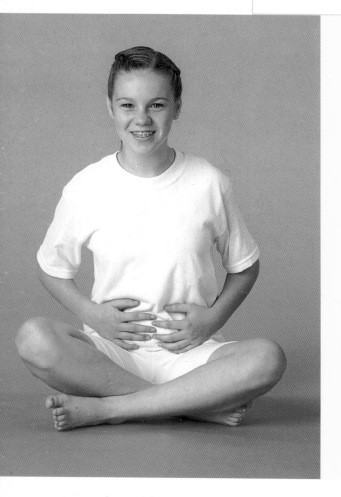

Elements

This breathing pose is a really good belly toner, and an excellent third chakra pose (see page 106). It's also excellent for aiding your child's elimination system, especially for constipation. Only do this breath on an empty stomach.

If you get lightheaded, it's just because you're getting more oxygen than you're used to. Breathe in and out normally and rest.

Awesome Anatomy

Our intestines absorb nutrients from our food into our bodies. Dragon Breath helps us clean the walls of the intestines. It loosens undigested particles that can clog things up, and helps move them out. The intestines are about 20 feet long, but they are coiled up so they can fit inside our bodies.

Musical Musings

As you snort in the Dragon Breath, use different rhythms. Snort fast. Snort slow. In musical terms, *staccato* means faster. *Adagio* means slower. Mix up your *adagio* and *staccato* Dragon Breaths—make a pattern and play your belly like a musical instrument.

Laughing Language

The yoga word *prana* means energy, vitality, life force. When you practice breaths like the dragon, which make you feel awake and alive, that is the *prana* at work.

Hot Air Balloon

Sit on your heels and inflate your balloon. Take little sips of breaths, as in Bunny Breath, and raise your arms upward little by little until they are over your head. When you've sipped in as much air as you can, your balloon is filled.

The first hot air balloon went up into the sky over southern France, about 200 years ago. In it were a sheep, a duck and a chicken. They flew for eight minutes.

Elements

For very young children, this pose is a great introduction to breathing. Our lungs fill like balloons when we breathe in (inhale) and deflate or empty when we breathe out (exhale).

Inflate your balloons together. Time it so you fill up at the same time. Fly around together in a hot-air-balloon dance and then deflate in a gentle heap. How many times can you go up, up, and away, and come back down?

We All Win/Awesome Anatomy

You will need three people to play "Balloon, Balloon." Fill real balloons. Rub them to make them stick to your body. Take turns giving directions like: Pass the balloon with your armpits (or wrists, or quadriceps, or sacrum). Say the name of the body part as you pass the balloon. Take turns being the caller.

See pages 104–105 for an anatomy chart.

Laughing Language

If an "in" breath is an inhalation, couldn't an "out" breath be an *out*halation? It makes perfect sense to us. Try to think of other original words we could invent.

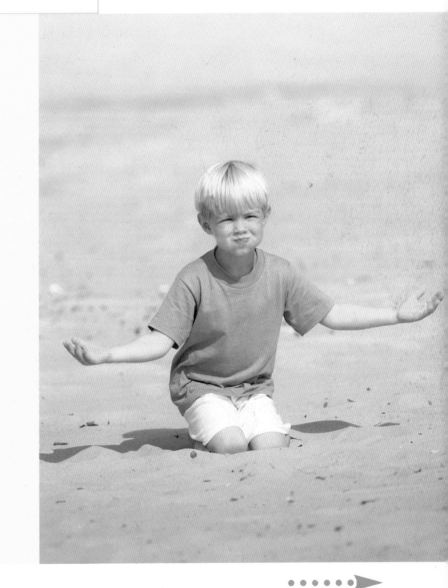

Hot Air Balloon (continued)

Bring your hands over your head to show the balloon expanding.

Get up and fly around.

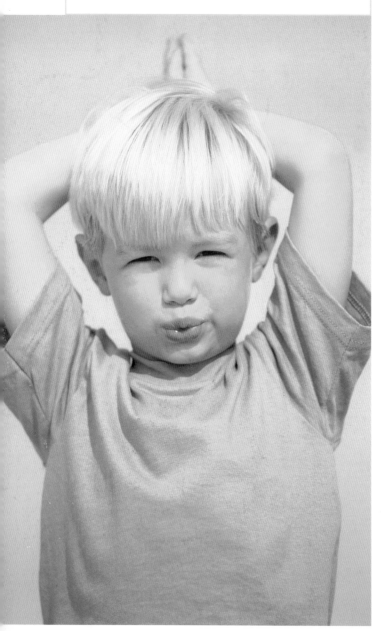

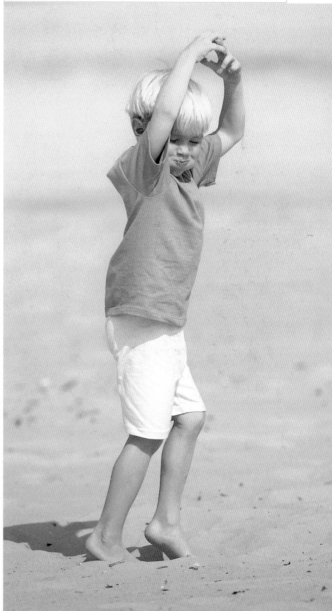

To land your balloon, blow out through your mouth and empty your lungs. Make noises like air escaping and collapse on the ground like an empty balloon.

Fall into Child's Pose (page 33) as you collapse. Rest. When you're ready, pump up your balloon again. Where will you fly this time?

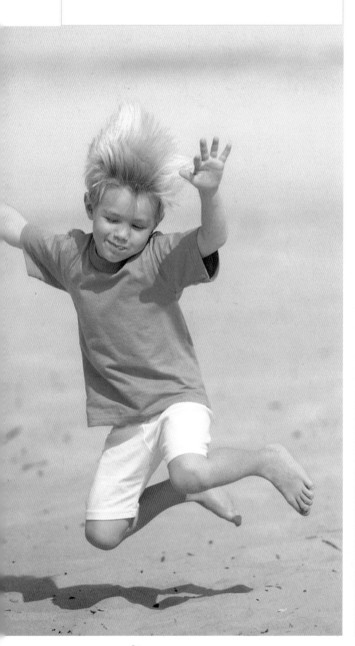

Butterfly with Antenna

When it emerges from its cocoon, a butterfly will rest on a twig and spread its wings to dry. Then it gently flaps its wings before taking its first flight. This pose is like a butterfly's flight.

Begin in L Sitting pose (page 20). Bring the bottoms of your feet together, with your heels close to your body. Open your knees out to each side. Stretch your neck and the top of your head toward the sky and make your spine longer. Place your hands at the sides of your head and stick up your pointer fingers to make antennae. Pull your arms back—now they're your wings. Breathe in and out as you flap your wings forward and back. Flap your leg wings up and down, too.

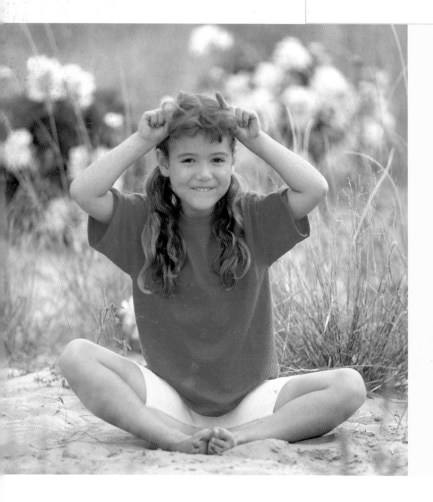

Elements
Children usually have a "sixth sense," or intuition, which often fades as they grow up. Whether you call it a hunch or gut feeling, help your child learn to trust it.

Ecological Echoes
Butterflies use their antennae the same way reptiles use their tongues. They are sense organs to detect danger and to get a general reading on things in the air.

Quiet Quests
Have you ever "just known" something even though you couldn't explain how you knew it? Maybe your antennae (your intuition) sensed it.

Laughing Language
Take a butterfly journey from A to Z. Think of a place that begins with the letter A. Fly there right away. Then think of a B place and fly there. Fly all the way to Zanzibar.

Brain Balance
Flapping your leg wings and your arm wings takes coordination and communication between the brain and the body.

Child's Pose

Begin in Heel Sitting pose (page 20). Open your knees a little, so your belly relaxes between your thighs. Bend at the hips and fold forward, letting your shoulders drop down, away from your ears and spine. Your arms lie back along the sides of your legs with open palms facing upward. Place your forehead on the floor, or turn it to one side for a while and then to the other side to gently stretch the neck. Take at least five breaths on each side.

Extended Child Pose: This time, lengthen your arms forward in front of you with palms facing downward. The Extended Child's Pose (see page 85) "extends" the spine, shoulders, arms and fingers. You can stay in either variation of the Child's Pose for as long as you want to.

This pose goes by many names in yoga. Sometimes we call it Acorn. Most call it the Child's Pose, because babies often sleep this way.

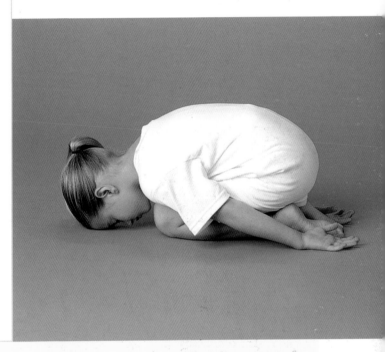

Elements
Any pose where you bend the body in half at the hips is a forward bend. Polar Bear (page 77) and Peanut Butter & Jelly (pages 92–93) are some examples. Forward bends are calming and quieting. Encourage your child to rest in the Child's Pose if she's feeling agitated.

Awesome Anatomy
Can you feel your ribs separating and moving as you breathe? Your intercostal muscles are at work. We call this breathing into your back.

Quiet Quests
Imagine a giant zipper from your neck to your tailbone. Use your breath to unzip it slowly from top to bottom. As it unzips, feel both sides of your back melt away from your spine. Breathe into your back. Let your back soften from your breath so that it feels boneless.

Ecological Echoes
Animals without backbones are called invertebrates. Some examples of invertebrates are worms and jellyfish. This pose might be renamed the Jellyfish pose.

Eyes Around the Clock

Just like the rest of the body, the eyes have muscles. These movements will exercise your eyes and make them stronger.

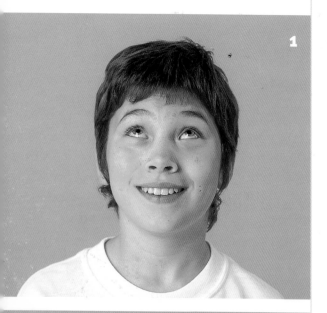

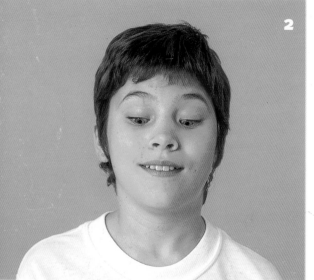

Take any seated position. Rub your hands together until they feel hot, then place the palms of your hands over your eyes and let them soak up the heat. Keep your fingers close together so no light comes through. You can keep your eyes closed or open. Use this technique in between the exercises to soothe and rest your eyes.

Imagine a clock hanging in front of your eyes. Repeating each direction six times, move your eyes to each position around the clock like this:

1 & 2: Look up and down, from twelve o'clock to six o'clock and from six o'clock to twelve o'clock.

3 & 4: Look right to left from three o'clock to nine o'clock and left to right from nine o'clock to three o'clock.

5 & 6: Look diagonally from one o'clock to seven o'clock and from seven o'clock to one o'clock. Then look from eleven o'clock to five o'clock and from five o'clock to eleven o'clock.

Now start at twelve o'clock and look at each number around the face of the clock. Then start again at twelve o'clock and move in the opposite direction. Circle the clock, clockwise, three times, then reverse. Try to keep your head still and move only your eyes.

Elements

If your child wears glasses, have her remove them for this exercise. In the beginning, the eye muscles might feel tired and sore. With practice, they'll feel more rested and alert.

When your child finishes the eye exercises she can move to her ears. Start at the top of the ear and gently squeeze or massage down the curl of the outer ear to the lobe, and back up. Do at least three rounds on each ear. This is a great way to bring your child's attention to her ears when she is not listening.

Visual Vignettes

Sharpen time-telling skills with this pose: Draw a clock with a round face, and put the numbers on in the correct places. Hang your clock on a wall in front of your child at eye level, or place it on the floor one or two feet in front of her.

Brain Balance

This pose links all the parts of our brain. It stimulates the corpus callosum, the brain's superhighway, which shuttles information back and forth.

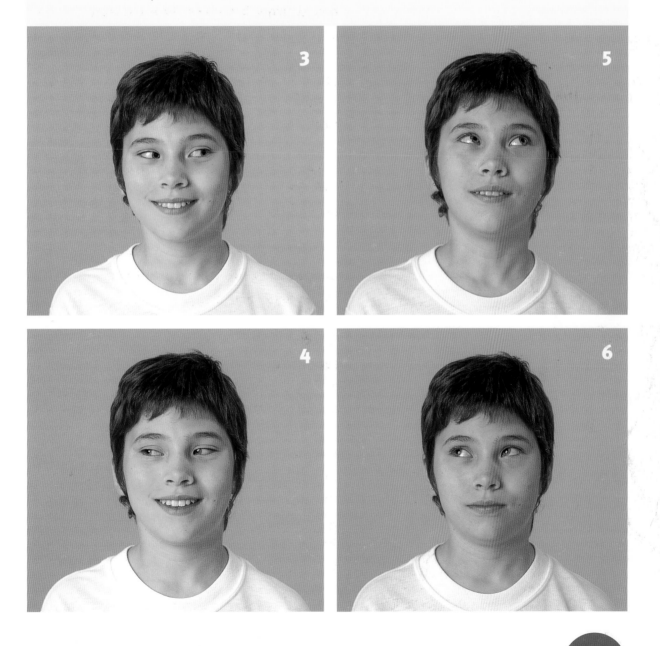

Tarzan's Thymus Tap

Gorillas do it. So do Tarzan and George of the Jungle. Why? Because it's fun, and it gives you energy and vitality.

Start in any of the base poses (page 20). Make two fists and pound your chest. Pound and tap under your arms, too. Howl and yowl and yodel. Feel the power and vibration of your sounds.

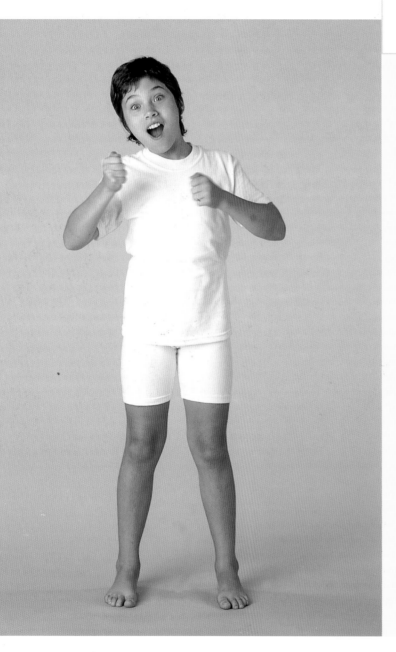

Elements

Try this exercise when your child is tired or cranky. Stimulating the thymus gland sends the flow of blood through the carotid arteries to the brain. It's a great pick-me-up.

Awesome Anatomy

Feel the collar bone (clavicle) that runs from shoulder to shoulder across the base of your throat. From the center of the clavicle draw a line down your chest. This is your breast bone (sternum). Run the fingers along your ribs. Gently tap these bones and the ribs. Don't forget to stimulate your armpits and the sides of your chest. They contain many important lymph glands.

Brain Balance

Tap all over your skull too, to energize the three parts of your brain.

1. The largest part, the main shape of the brain, is the cerebrum. It allows us to feel, think, sense, and learn.
2. The brain stem, near the top of the neck, controls the body functions that we don't need to think about because they just happen, like breathing and our heartbeat.
3. The cerebellum, or mini-brain, is at the back of the brain, behind the brain stem. It plays a key part in posture and balance and acts like an "automatic pilot" when we ride a bicycle, use a keyboard, or drive.

Pedal Laughing

Lie on your back. Bend your arms and legs like you're riding a bicycle in the air. Pedal forward: laugh. Pedal backward: laugh. It might be hard to really laugh at first, but once you get started, you won't be able to stop. Have fun and be silly with this one.

People say that laughter is the best medicine. Laughter is a language that all people speak and understand. So go ahead—laugh, pedal, and feel great!

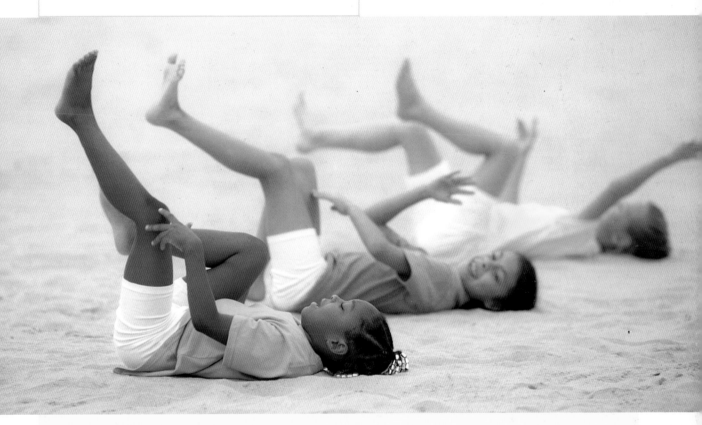

Elements

When was the last time you and your child laughed together? Try it, especially when you're not connecting, and feel the barriers melt away. Great guffaws feel good!

Laughter lowers blood pressure, reduces stress hormones, increases muscle flexion, boosts immune function, and produces endorphins—a natural high.

Bridge of Diamonds

Laughing is a bonding experience. In India there are laughing clubs, where people gather for one purpose—to laugh together.

Musical Musings

Form a Pedal Laughing chorus. High-tone laughers are sopranos and lower ones are bass. Medium-low laughers are tenors and medium-high are altos.

Moo and Meow

The bones that make up the spine are called vertebrae. Humans have 26 vertebrae, while cats and cows have about 52. This pose keeps your spine flexible.

Begin in All Fours (page 20). Line up your wrists under your shoulders. Spread your fingers wide and arch your spine to the sky. Loosen your neck and drop your head down. Breathe out long and catlike as you meoooooowwwwww.

Now lift your chest forward and look up with big cow eyes. Dip your belly down and tilt your sit bones (your ischium) up. Your back will sink down like a cow's. Make cow lips and moo deeply from the back of your throat. Mooooooo. Go back and forth, meowing and mooing. Feel the cat change into a cow and back into a cat. Begin with four rounds. Increase one round at a time.

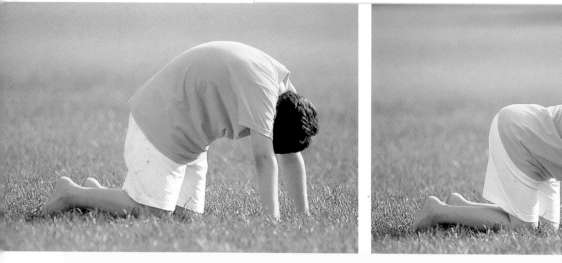

Elements

This simple pose has so many benefits. It stretches the front and back of the body and frees the neck and head. It improves the suppleness and strength of the spine. Do the Moo and Meow every day to keep backaches at bay.

Math Medley

The arched cat back is a convex curve; that is, it curves outward instead of inward. The cow spine is concave, so the curve is inward, not outward. A scoop of ice cream is convex, but the inside of the cone is concave. Maybe that's why they're so good together!

Visual Vignettes/Laughing Language

Some convex shapes are baseball caps, camels, domes of buildings, and Wheel pose. Some concave shapes are skating ramps, bowls, funnels, and Row Your Boat pose. Find these different shapes in your house or outdoors. Draw and label them.

Lizard

Lie on your belly. Place your hands under your shoulders. Spread your fingers out like lizard claws. Bend your lizard toes forward. Push up until your arms and legs are straight. Draw your shoulders back and away from your ears. Walk like a lizard, slowly and carefully. Flick your tongue in and out as you check for danger and maybe catch a bug for a snack. Your scales protect you and will keep you strong and fearless.

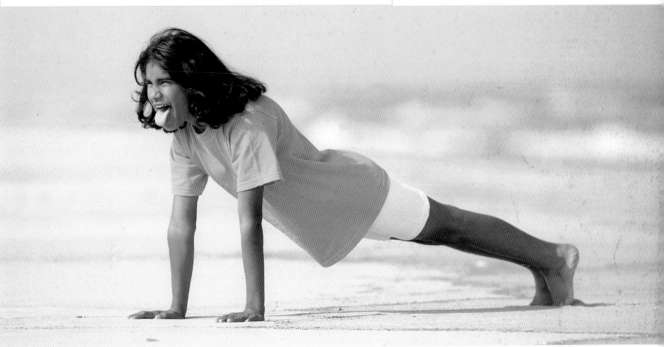

Elements

Lizard can also be practiced in a stationary position, but kids really like to scurry and have lizard races.

If you or your child suffers from TMJD (temporomandibular joint disorder) or grind your teeth, practicing lizard tongue will help. Clenching the jaw sends signals of tightness to the brain via the sensory nerves. The motor nerves then communicate that sense back to the body.

Laughing Language
Make tongue-twisters with the letter *L*, such as "Long lizards lie lollygagging."

We All Win
Take a lizard walk with a partner while you trade tongue-twisters.

Math Medley
How far can you walk as a lizard? Count your stepss.

39

Down Diggety Doggy Down

Dogs have been our best friends for over 12,000 years. They frequently roam in packs, the way many kids and teens like to do. This is a tough pose, but it will make you feel down-diggety-doggy good!

Elements

This pose strengthens the legs and arms and relieves stiffness in the shoulders. It can also help correct curvature of the spine (scoliosis).

Children love to "walk" their parents, so try this role-reversal activity (see photo 4).

Math Medley/Musical Musings/We All Win

Play the Canine Calling game. One child creates a pattern of growls, barks, and other doglike sounds. The other child repeats it, and adds more sounds. Go back and forth.

Awesome Anatomy

This pose works the muscles of the legs—ankles, calves, and hamstrings. (See Awesome Anatomy, page 104.) When you first do this pose, your leg muscles might feel really tight, but with time and practice they will grow stronger and more elastic.

1. Begin on your hands and knees in All Fours (page 20).

2. Bend your toes forward. Spread your fingers wide. Press your doggy paws and heels downward as you lift your hips and tail to the sky. Lengthen your spine. Stretch your arms and legs as long as possible. Let your head hang down. Growl, yawn, bark, and make other doggy sounds.

3. Bend your knee and rotate your belly and chest upward. Raise one leg up and "mark your territory" just like dogs do. Keep your hands pressing downward and your arms straight. Dogs leave their scent so other animals know they've been there. Lift your opposite leg too.

4. Take turns "walking the dog." Grab the back of the "dog's" shirt like you're holding a leash. Lead him around. Give him directions; slower, faster, turn around.

Let your doggy rest after the walk. Have her lie on her back with her arms and legs in the air. Scratch her behind her ears. Scratch her belly too. Give her a bone and a kiss on her nose before she rolls over and stretches back into Down Diggety Doggy Down.

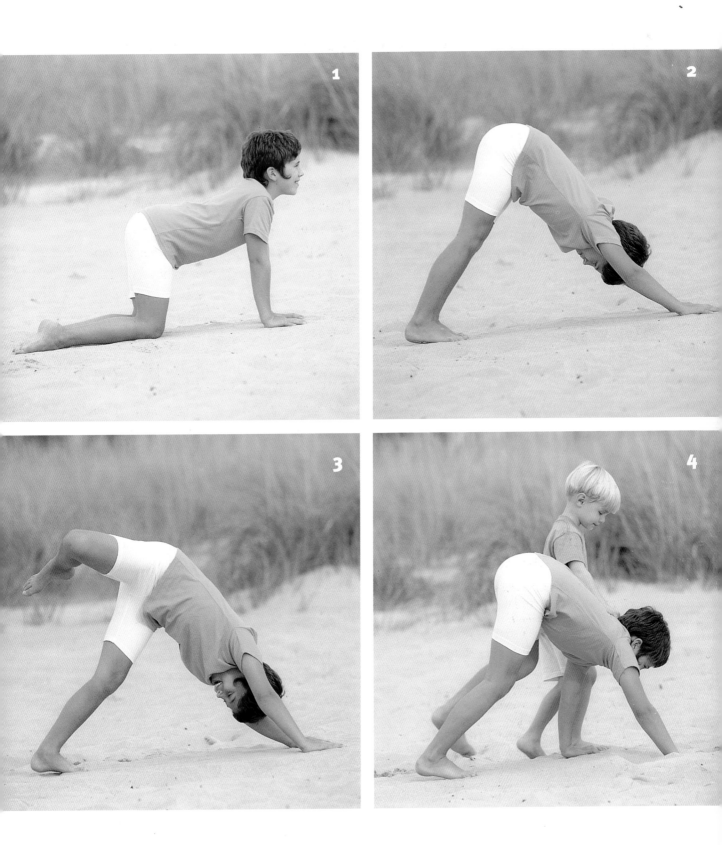

Dromedary Delight

The Bactrian camel has two humps; another type of camel, the dromedary, has only one. Both store fat (not water) in their humps.

Kneel on the floor with your legs and knees hip-width apart. Press the tops of your feet into the floor, push your thighs forward, bring your hands to your lower back, fingers pointing upward, and lift your chest. Breathe evenly in and out as you extend your rib cage and broaden your chest.

Continue to lift your chest with each breath as you curl your toes forward and bring your hands to your heels to imitate the camel's hump. Your head can fall back (as shown) or tuck into your chest.

Delight in the dromedary for ten seconds. Rest in the Child's Pose (page 33) after each of these backbends. Repeat. Increase the duration and repetitions of the pose as your spine and chest become more flexible.

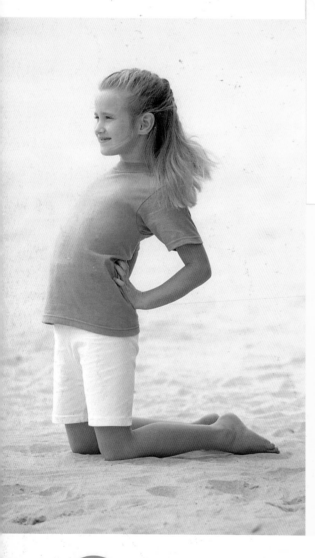

Elements

This pose strengthens the back and kidneys. Because of its chest-opening ability, it can increase lung capacity and is especially beneficial for children with asthma. It also helps the posture of those with drooping shoulders and rounded backs.

Bactrian camels and dromedaries are said to spit when they are angry and make *tissskkkk* sounds. Invite your child to please be a delightful dromedary—make the sound, but hold the spit.

Ecological Echoes

Dromedaries avoid trotting and galloping to save water and energy. They can survive for months without water and can drink up to 35 gallons of water at a time.

Awesome Anatomy

The lungs are light and spongy and are filled with millions of air channels, which provide an enormous surface to absorb oxygen. If your lungs were unfolded, they'd make a slippery surface the size of a tennis court!

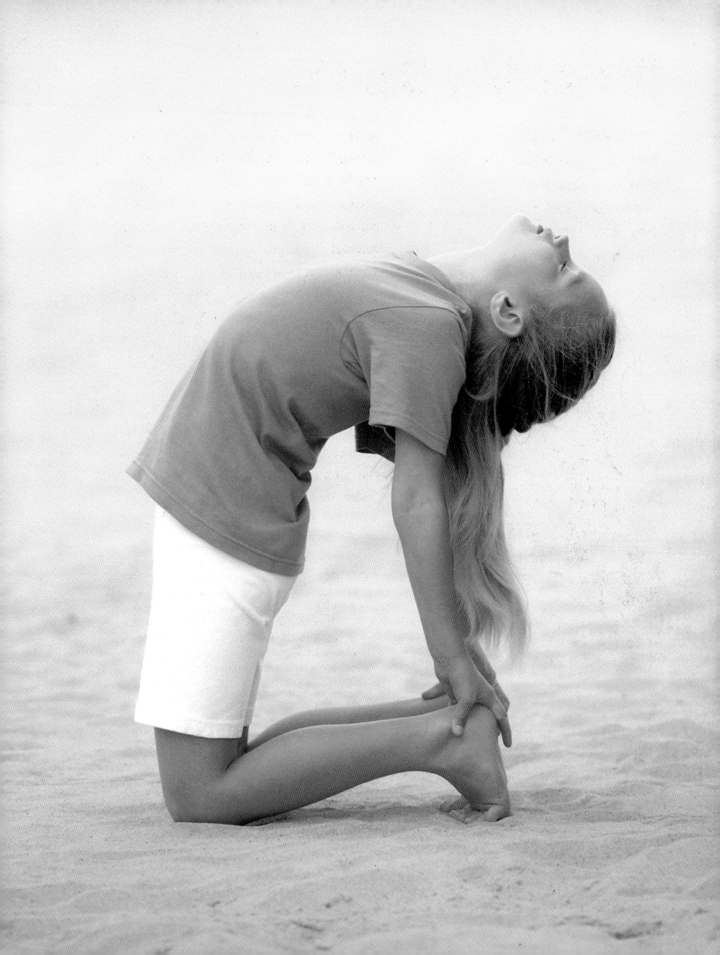

Untying the Knots

Does your body ever feel like it's been tied in knots? Well, loosen up, untie, shake, flop, and relax.

Untie your neck. Roll your head around. Untie your shoulders. Move them up, down, all around. Untie all your knotted muscles and joints from head to toe. Massage and stroke them after you've untied them. Untie till you feel nice and loose—like a goose or a moose without a noose!

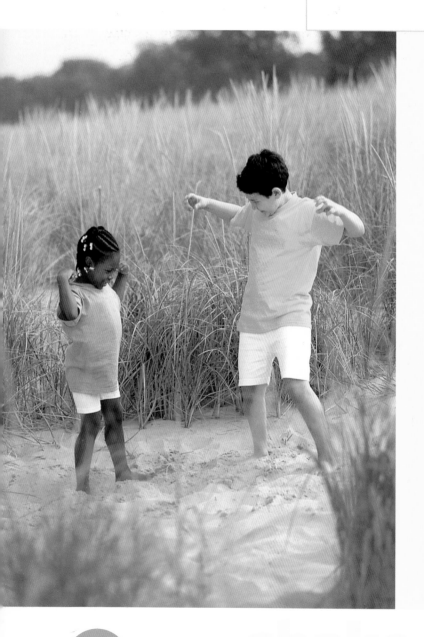

Elements

We know what it feels like to be tied in knots. Children do, too. Many times, though, they can't express how they feel without lashing out. These poses are a great way to help them let their yucky feelings out in expressive ways.

Feelings and emotions are in the realm of the second chakra (see page 106). Talk about the differences between feeling like you're all tied in knots and being loose as a goose. Being loose produces those brain hormones, endorphins, which work like magic to help us feel good.

Awesome Anatomy

As you untie each muscle or joint, say its name. Look at page 104 to find the names of many parts of your body.

Musical Musings

Put on some moving and grooving music. (See page 114 for recommendations.) Untie. Shake. Flop. Play Freeze and Flow— when the music stops, freeze. When the music starts again, flow.

We All Win

Tangle a part of your body around a part of another person. Entwine arms, legs, toes, or fingers. See how twisted you can get. Slowly, gently, and peacefully untangle. Then hang forward and hang out in Ragdoll.

Shake Like Jelly

Now shake like jelly. Shake all over. Go crazy. Jiggle, wiggle, and giggle. You know how.

Ragdoll Ann and Ragdoll Andy

Now that you're untied and jellified, hang out in a forward bend. Breathe in and feel your whole body lighten. Breathe out and fold yourself in half, bending from the hips. Do you feel like Ragdoll Ann or Andy? Loosen your neck and let your head and arms hang down, soft and squishy just like a rag doll. To come up, place your hands on your tailbone and inch your fingers up your spine, feeling the bumpy vertebrae as you slowly straighten back up to standing.

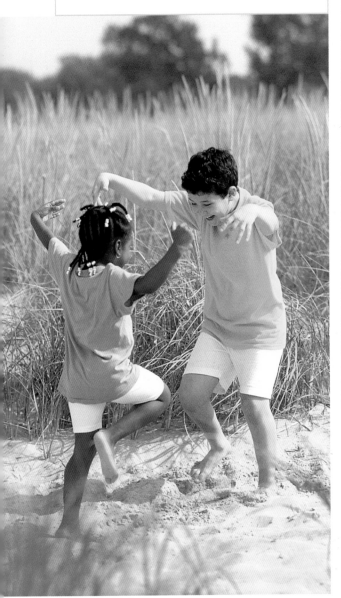

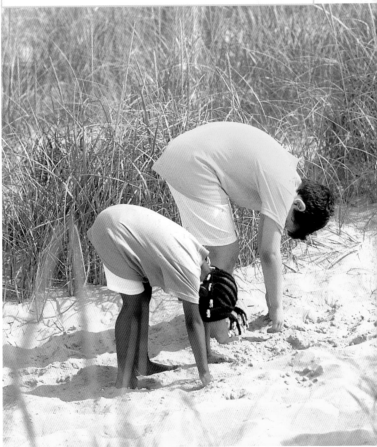

shake like jelly

45

Bow and Arrow

Focus as you pull your bowed leg back and release your arrow skyward.

Begin in L Sitting pose (page 20). Bend your right knee. Grab the big toe of your right foot with your right fingers. Put your left hand flat on the floor alongside your hip and use that arm to support your spine and chest. Keep your spine tall. Breathe in as you pull your bent leg back behind you. Breathe out with a *whoosh* sound and shoot your leg *across* the opposite leg. Do this six times, then change sides.

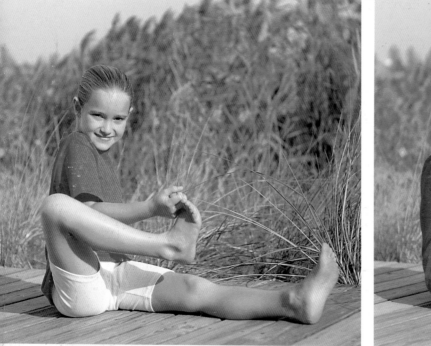
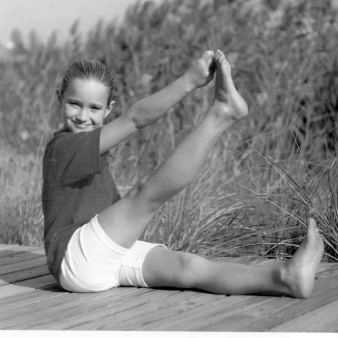

Elements
Many children shoot the leg straight ahead or out to the side instead of shooting across. But the crossover movement stimulates brain communication.

Math Medley/Visual Vignettes
Notice the lines, angles, and shapes your arms and legs take as you launch and shoot your bow and arrow. Does your leg triangle get bigger or smaller the more you are able to cross over? Draw the shape of your leg triangle.

Awesome Anatomy
Bow and Arrow opens the hips and lengthens the hamstrings, as well as the gastrocnemius and soleus muscles of the lower leg.

Twist and Blow

Lie on your back, knees bent, and stretch your arms out to each side, in line with your shoulders, palms up. Drop your bent knees over to the right, and up towards the armpits. Turn your head to the left as you breathe out, with a blowing sound. Breathe in and bring your knees back to the center and across your belly. Drop your legs to the left side, turn your head to the right, and breathe out. Do five continuous rounds. Then relax for at least a minute with your knees on one side and head rotated in the opposite direction. Change sides and relax again.

This pose is a spine-twister! It soothes, stretches, and strengthens the back and belly at the same time.

Elements

This pose gives the kidneys, liver, stomach, and intestines an inner massage. The twisting action that takes place revitalizes the spine while improving the digestive and eliminative systems.

Math Medley/Awesome Anatomy

Your spinal cord runs inside the spine from the base of the brain to the tip of the back. There are 24 individual and 2 fused vertebrae (see if you can count them). There are 31 pairs of spinal nerves that branch out from there and connect to every part of the body.

Brain Balance

The base of the spine is called the sacrum. The top of the head is called the cranium. This twisting pose stimulates the spine, the central nervous system, and its control center, the brain.

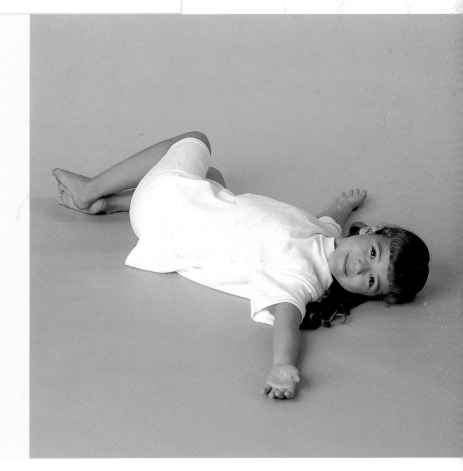

Eagle

**Perch with your lower body.
Fly with your upper body.**

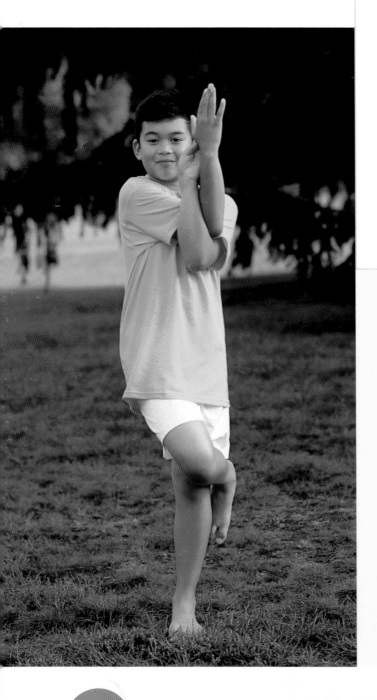

Begin in Mountain pose (page 49). Bring your bent arms up in front of you and place the left elbow on top of the right. Twist together your forearms and press your palms together in Namaste position. You can also interlace your fingers. Bend your knees. Lift your left leg and wrap it over your right leg, as in the picture. If you can, hide your left foot and toes behind your right calf. Untangle yourself and change sides. Try to balance for 10 seconds on each side and gradually increase the time. Use a focus friend if you need guidance.

Elements

The entwining of the arms and hands is a great stretch for the upper back and shoulders, as well as the fingers and wrist joints. If your child spends a considerable amount of time at the computer, have her take Eagle breaks periodically to prevent hunched shoulders. She can do Half Eagle without even getting up from the computer. This is a good idea for you, too.

Ecological Echoes

Eagles can glide great distances without flapping their wings. Their wings contain about 7,000 feathers and are aerodynamically perfect. Known for their keen eyesight, eagles can see fish in the water from hundreds of feet up in the air, or spot a rabbit moving a mile away.

Brain Balance

The twisting of the arms and legs in this refreshing and invigorating balance pose infuses the spine and increases blood flow to the brain.

Mountain

Stand tall and proud,
strong and majestic,
just like a mountain.

1. Stand with your feet together or hip-width apart, whichever is most comfortable. Arms are at your sides, fingers stretching toward the floor.

2. Tell your toes: *Big toes stay on the floor, others lift up* (left). Now tell them: *Big toes lift up, all others stay on the floor* (right). Tell your heels to lift, and put them back down (center).

Press your feet into the ground. This downward action through the legs allows the torso, neck and head to rise like a mountain above the clouds. Notice how tall and light you feel.

Elements
This pose can help improve posture and correct flat feet, as well as improve the ability to stand still and steady.

Quiet Quests
Feel your breath moving through your Mountain body, upward and downward from the earth to the sky. We are the conduits of this natural flow and exchange of energy. Take 3 to 5 breaths. Increase with practice.

Laughing Language
Tell or write a story as if you really were a mountain. Add lots of details.

Brain Balance
With time and practice the toes will respond to the brain's directions more easily. Our 10 billion brain cells can make over 10 trillion connections. With yoga, new pathways, or axons, are being formed all the time.

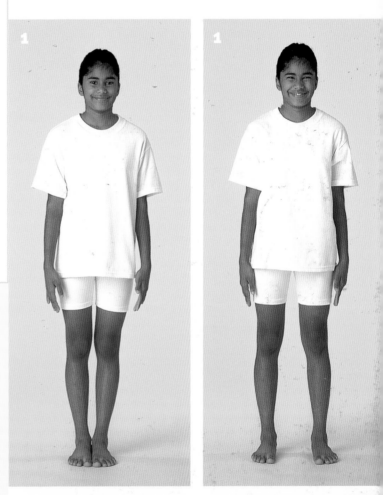

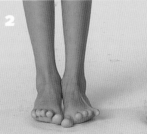

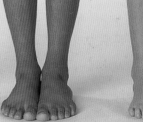

Volcano

When you feel like bursting or exploding, use Volcano to let off steam in a peaceful way.

Begin in Mountain pose (page 49).
Bring the fingertips together
at the chest.

Elements

Parents tell us that children use this technique when they feel angry or frustrated. Encourage them to release feelings and emotions in this safe way.

Ecological Echoes

Volcanoes look like mountains, and may erupt when they get too hot. Lava is melted rock that bursts out of volcanoes. We use the Volcano pose to release "steam," too!

Math Medley

In the last 10,000 years 1,511 volcanoes have erupted, not including tens of thousands of volcanoes on the sea floor. Can you write out those numbers? Figure the average number of eruptions each year. (Hint: Divide the years by the number of volcanoes.)

Laughing Language

YogaKids imagine surprising things inside their volcanoes: feelings, food, and toys are just a few categories. Here are some examples:

> My volcano is filled with lollipops.
> My volcano is filled with angry steam.
> My volcano is filled with kittens.

Name all the things that are released from your volcano as you practice.

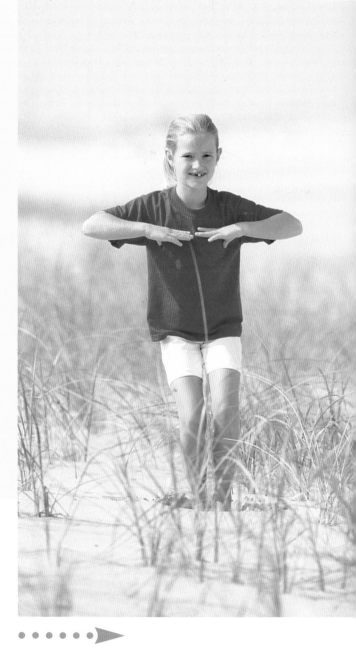

Jump the feet apart.

Place your palms together at the center of your body (Namaste position).

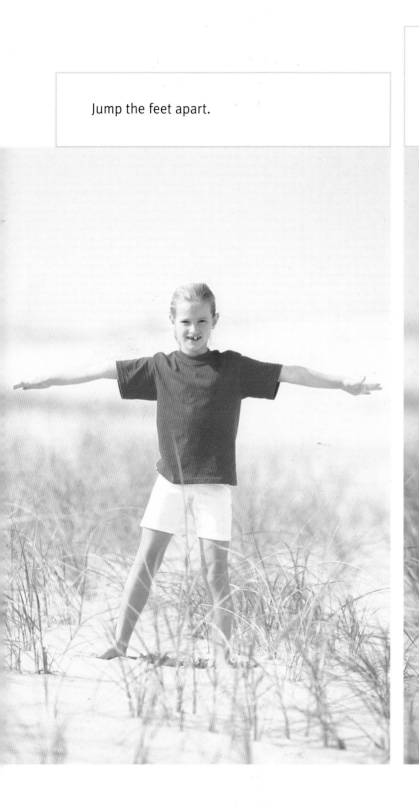

Volcano (continued)

Breathe in. Watch your hands as you raise them over your head.

Breathe out as you explode your arms outward.

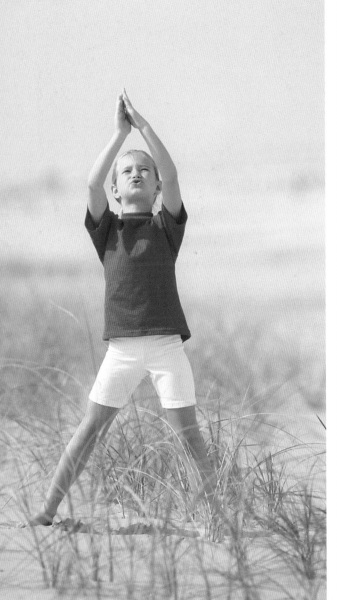

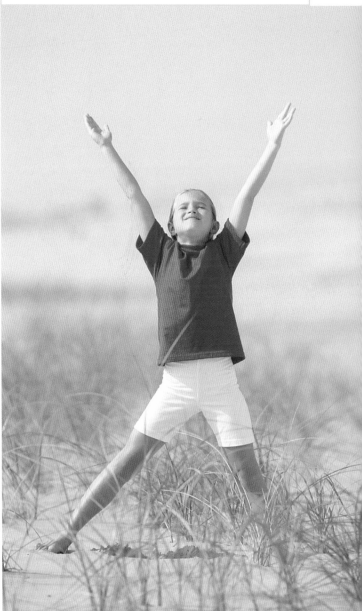

Lower them to your sides and return your hands to Namaste.

Erupt and release again and again. Make big, exploding-volcano noises.

Jump your feet back together when you're finished erupting.

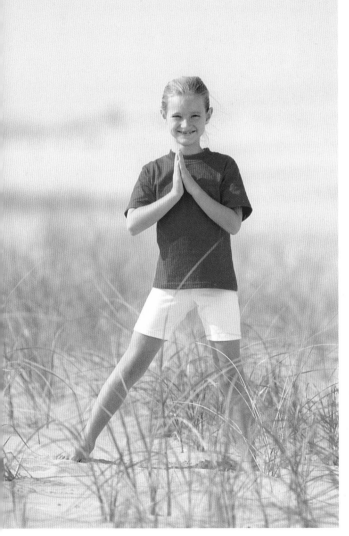

Warrior Series

A true warrior is strong without weapons. A warrior's mind is sharp and focused. You are a warrior. You have inner strength and determination.

Right Angle   Obtuse Angle   Acute Angle

There are three basic variations of the Warrior pose. In YogaKids we practice them in the following sequence:

Brave Warrior

Begin by jumping your feet apart (page 20). Turn both feet to the right (for feet details, see page 88). Try to bend your right knee into a right angle so your thigh is almost parallel to the ground—that is, as level as a tabletop. Stretch out your arms. Turn your head to the right. Focus at a spot somewhere past your fingers. Say, "I am brave."

Elements

The Warrior series will increase stamina and flexibility in the legs, arms, shoulders, and back. Each of these poses can be practiced by itself or in the series.

Math Medley

A right angle is 90 degrees.
An obtuse angle is greater than 90 degrees.
An acute angle is less than 90 degrees.
Try to feel or see these in the Warrior poses.

Affirmations

It often helps to say out loud the things you want to feel or do in your life. That's really what an affirmation is. For example, if you are sick, try saying, "I am feeling better." If you are nervous about a test, try, "I am smart," or "I will ace this." See page 111 for more affirmations.

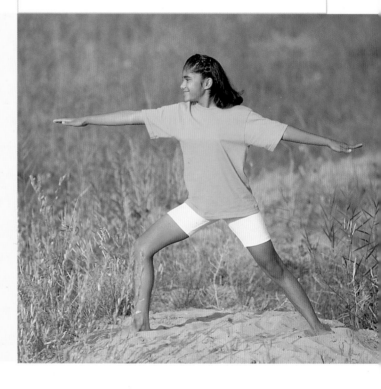

Bold Warrior

Turn your hips toward your right leg, keeping the leg bent. Raise your arms straight above your head. Say, "I am bold."

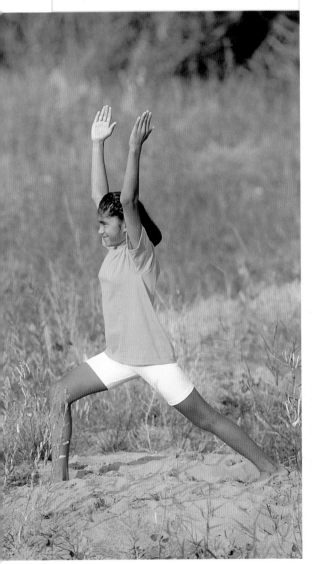

Powerful Warrior

Then shift your weight onto your right leg. Pick up your left foot and leg and stretch it back behind you. Keep both legs as straight and strong as possible. Stretch your arms forward. Say, "My own power I can hold."

Now do all the steps again in reverse order. Bring your left leg back down, bend your right knee, and repeat Bold Warrior. Turn your upper body forward and stretch your arms out to the side. Repeat Brave Warrior. Turn your feet to the left and repeat the Warrior series on the left side.

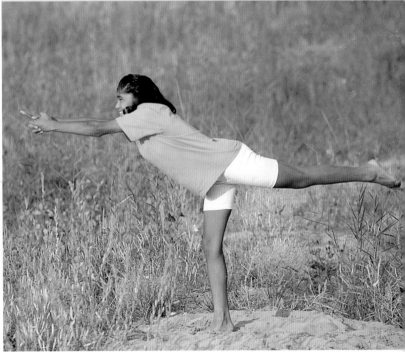

Tree

Trees are our best friends: They give us the oxygen we need, and we give them back the carbon dioxide they need.

Begin in Mountain pose (page 49). Lift your right foot, bend your right knee, and press your foot against the inside of your left leg. You can use your hand to place your foot anywhere between your ankle and inner thigh. As your balance gets stronger, you'll be able to raise your foot higher up your leg.

Bring your hands to your chest, palms together in Namaste position, then raise your arms up above your head. Stretch them out wide, like the branches of a tree. Separate your fingers. Balance for three breaths in and out. Increase as you're ready.

Practice Tree on the left side. Use a focus friend if you need help with this pose.

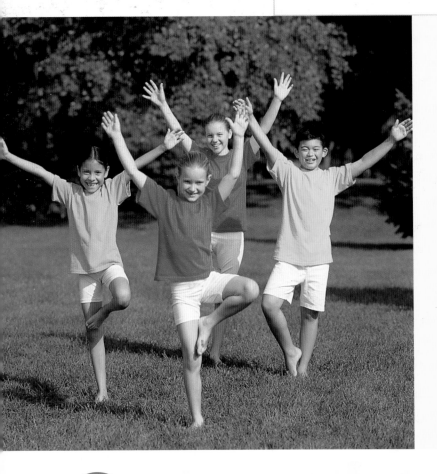

Elements

The Tree pose fosters balance and concentration, as well as strengthening the shoulders and legs. To succeed in balance poses, let go of your thoughts. Connect with the rhythm of your breath.

Awesome Anatomy/Ecological Echoes

Your body is like a tree. Your feet are the roots, and your legs and torso are the trunk. Your outstretched arm and finger branches provide homes for bird's nests, playgrounds for squirrels and chipmunks, and perches for jaguars and panthers to lounge on.

We All Win

Play Wind in the Trees: One person is the tree, another person the wind. The wind blows on the tree and tries to knock it over. The tree stands rooted and strong and tries to withstand the wind. When you have a whole forest of trees, as in the photo, this game is really fun.

Flamingo

Begin in Mountain pose (page 49). Spreading your arms open like graceful wings, extend your left leg straight back. Bend forward at the hips. Establish your balance little by little, adjusting your arms and back leg. Clear your mind and fix your attention on your breath, your body, or a focus friend. You will notice that when your thoughts are scattered, your pose is unsteady. If you feel like flying, gently flap your wings. Repeat with the opposite leg. Do both sides 2 or 3 times.

The word flamingo comes from the Latin word for flame. Flamingos are born with soft gray feathers. Around their third birthday, their feathers turn flaming pink or orange. That's quite a birthday present!

Elements

Flamingo legs might look scrawny and spindly, but they're not. This pose strengthens, shapes, and tones the legs. Strong legs help the upper body feel feather-light. Praise your child as you see her become more graceful, poised, and balanced.

Ecological Echoes

A flamingo flies with its head and neck stretched out in front. And, unlike other feathered friends, flamingos bend and stretch their legs behind them when balancing. Can you feel the difference between Stork (page 59) and Flamingo?

Math Medley

Flamingo wings are about 60 inches from tip to tip. How many feet is that? (Hint: 1 foot = 12 inches.) What is your wingspan? Measure from fingertip to fingertip.

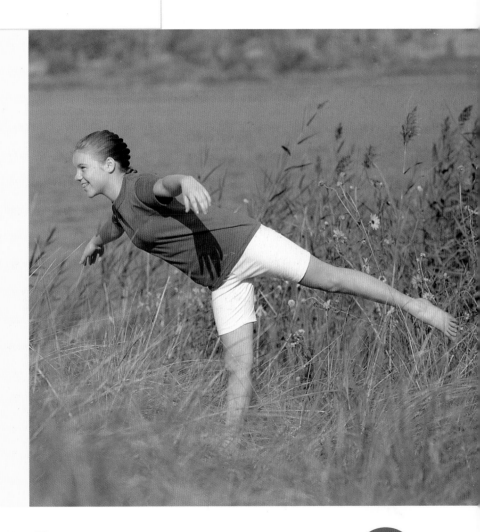

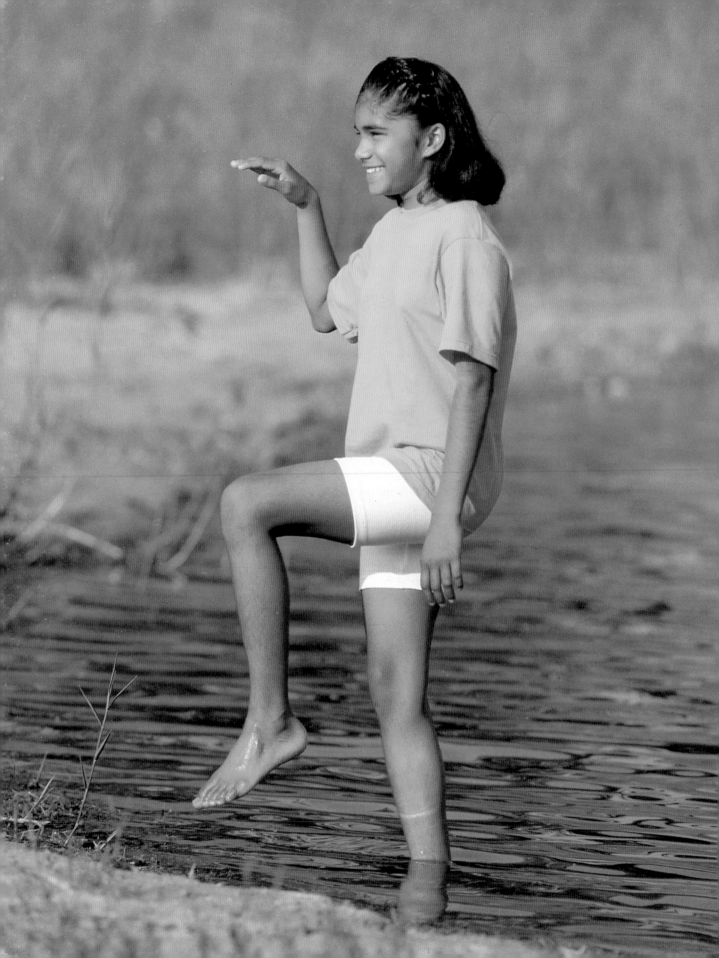

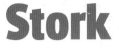

The stork is a symbol of good luck. Make a wish when you practice the Stork pose, and you might just get what you ask for.

Begin in Mountain pose (page 49). Breathe evenly in and out. Gaze at a focus friend to help you balance.

Bend your left knee and lift your left foot off the ground. Keep your leg at a right angle (left) or tuck your foot inside your knee (below).

Lift your right arm and bend it at the elbow. Relax your wrist. Begin by holding the pose for 5 seconds. With patience and practice, you'll stand steady and become an expert at this balancing act.

Elements
All of the YogaKids® Feathers poses are about balance. Stork is one of the easier ones, so it's a good place to begin. Balance poses help us learn stillness and focus, two important skills for both children and adults.

Ecological Echoes
Swamps and marshes are two of the stork's favorite restaurants. On the menu are insects, fish, frogs, reptiles, young birds, and small mammals. Do you eat some of the same foods as the stork?

Math Medley
Count the number of seconds you can hold your Stork pose. Try to hold your balance for a few more seconds each time you try. Soon you'll be up to a minute, or even 2 or 3 minutes. How many seconds is that? (Hint: 60 seconds = 1 minute.)

Bridge of Diamonds
Storks are loving and nurturing parents. The legend that the stork brings the new baby arises from the fact that they take very good care of their young.

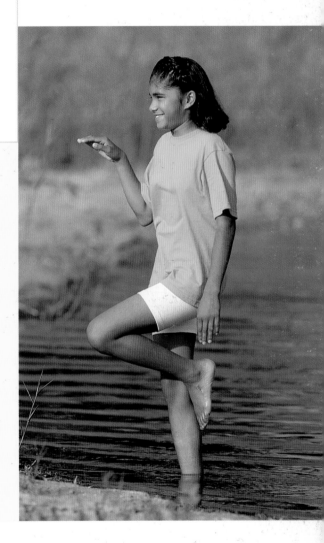

360-Degree Owl

Owls are known for their beauty and intelligence. Their amazing eyesight and hearing makes them great hunters too. They can't move their eyes, but they can turn their heads almost in a full circle.

Roll up your yoga mat and turn it into a tree branch. Bend your knees and perch on your branch. Find your balance and sit as upright as you can. Tuck your arms behind you. Hold each elbow with the opposite hand. Turn your head slowly from side to side, eyes wide open. Can you see what's behind you?

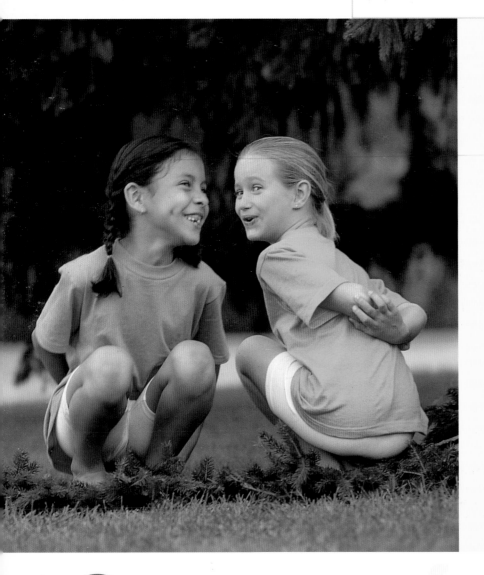

Elements

360-Degree Owl improves balance, posture, and flexibility in the joints, especially the neck, hips, knees, and ankles. And it's fun to inhabit another kind of animal for a short time.

Musical Musings

Owls can flap their wings silently and can hear even the tiniest sounds to find their prey. If you perch quietly in this pose for at least a minute, what tiny sounds can you hear?

Laughing Language

Many owl calls sound to us like human speech. The great horned owl seems to say, "Who's awake? Me, too!" The barred owl says, "Who cooks for you?" What would you say if you were an owl?

Visual Vignettes

Draw a picture of yourself with wings and feathers. What would it feel like to be a bird?

Crow

Begin in Open Mountain pose (page 49). Bend your knees and squat down. Place your arms to the inside of your bent legs and press your hands with outstretched fingers into the floor. Lean slightly forward. Bend your elbows outward to make a shelf for your knees. Rise onto your tiptoes and place your left knee on your left "arm shelf." Then carefully place your right knee on your right "arm shelf." In the beginning, you may only be able to lift one foot at a time off the floor. With patience and practice, you will balance in Crow. As you do, see if you can increase the time you can stay balanced.

Crows are very intelligent animals. Like parrots, they can be trained to mimic our voices. They are known for their good memories and their love of shiny objects.

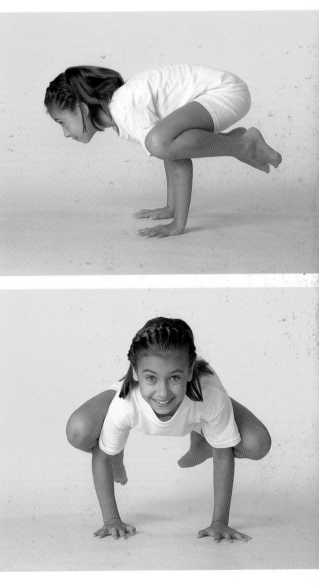

Elements

This is a difficult pose that requires strength and focus. It builds self-esteem and confidence and strengthens the arms. It even tones the belly, because the abdominal muscles automatically contract to help balance.

With children under five years old, getting up into the actual balance part of the pose is generally impossible. They can follow the instructions, however, and you can guide them in the steps to teach them patience and determination.

Musical Medley

Birds put on shows for each other, just like we do. To impress their mates, they put on dramatic flight shows, as well as bowing, strutting, and puffing their feathers as they perform. Can you imagine dancing in the Crow pose?

Ecological Echoes

Crows eat at the same restaurants as their feathered friends the storks. They are both *omnivorous*, which means that they eat plants as well as small animals. *Herbivores* eat only plants. *Carnivores* eat mainly other animals.

Electric Circle

Join hands and feel the energy we all share.

Elements

Our bodies are full of electricity. The heart is the power supply and the breath is the generator.

Awesome Anatomy

Your heart lies just left of center in your chest. Find your heartbeat. The muscle in your heart contracts around 100,000 times a day. The heart pumps blood all over the body.

Laughing Language

Amps, volts, and *watts*: those three words describe amounts of electric power, and all three come from the names of the scientists who first described them. Name your personal electricity after yourself—marshas or susies, for instance.

Bridge of Diamonds

The right side of the body is considered the male, or sun, side. The sun shines downward, so the right hand is down. The left side is considered the female, or moon, side. The moon reflects the light, so the left hand is turned up.

Do this pose with at least three people. Sit cross-legged with your hands on your knees. The left hand rests palm-up, and the right hand rests palm-down. Breathe deeply into your heart space at the center of your chest. Feel the breath move across the chest, flow down the arms and into the hands that you are holding. You might feel heat or tingling. Whenever you feel this electricity, gently squeeze the hands you're holding. That is the signal to let each other know that the circuit has been made and the current is flowing.

With your lips closed and your tongue curled upward to touch the roof of your mouth, start humming or buzzing to imitate the sound of electricity. Get louder and louder, then break the circuit by letting go of hands and releasing your tongue. Sit quietly and listen to the silence.

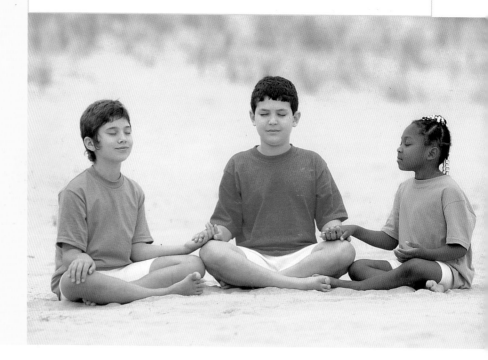

Sit and Twist

Sit cross-legged in front of your partner with your four knees touching. Put your right arm behind your back, reach out with your left hand and grab your partner's right hand. Breathe in and sit up tall. Breathe out, turn away from your partner, twist your spine, and look over your right shoulder. When you twist, rotate your spine gradually from the tip of your tail to the top of your head. Inhale as you lengthen your spine and exhale as you twist. Sit and twist for five breaths. Unfurl and change sides (left arm behind your back; right hand reaches across and grabs your partner's left hand). Sit and twist for five breaths in this way.

The word *yoga* means "to yoke" or "join." Try these partner poses to connect two and make one.

Elements

Partner poses are designed to help two people achieve greater mobility than either could alone. Partner poses work best when the partners are approximately the same size and weight, but that is not always possible. Have fun and encourage one another to stretch to your maximum and enjoy the partner play.

Talk to one another. For example, "Can you twist more?" or "That's too much pull for me." Teach your children to ask for what they need.

We All Win

Help each other twist and lengthen to your "edge." Going to your "edge" in yoga means that you practice the pose the best you can in the moment. Do not force or strain. Do keep breathing and moving as deeply as you can. Gently guide each other.

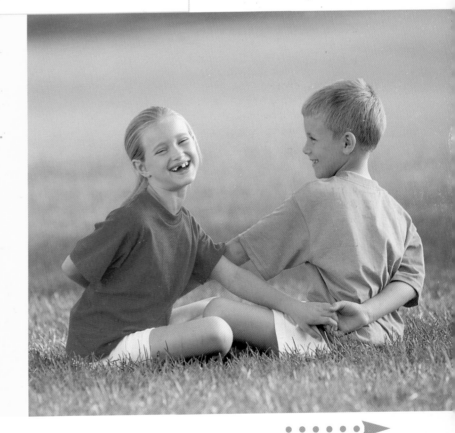

Rib-Splitting Seated Triangle

Sit with your legs wide apart in a triangle position. Flex your heels and bend your toes toward you. The person with the smaller triangle should press her heels into her partner's inner ankles. Reach across and take hold of your partner's right hand or wrist. Firmly plant your sit bones (your ischium) into the earth. Lift your left arm up above your head and over to the right as you stretch all the way through the fingertips. Feel the spaces created between the ribs. Lean away as you rotate your ribcage toward the sky. Look up. Bring your hand toward the opposite foot. Smile and breathe in and out. Come back to center. Change sides.

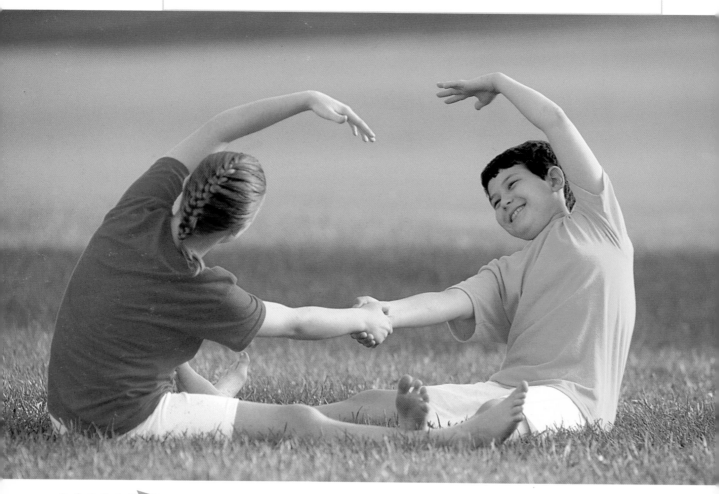

Seesaw Triangle

Remain in the Seated Triangle. Continue to press your
legs downward and flex your feet. Keep your sit bones
planted in the earth. Reach your arms straight across to
your partner and take hold of each other's wrists or
hands. As one person bends forward at the hip hinge, the
other leans back and gently guides her partner's upper
body forward. After a few breaths, switch the person
being pulled forward and the person leaning back. Gently
rock each other back and forth, like a seesaw.

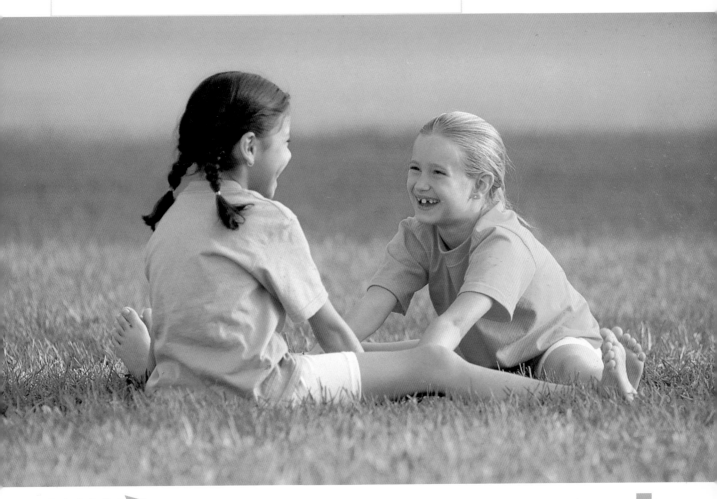

L Is for Left

L is for Love.
L is for Light.
L is for Left.

Sit down with your legs together and stretched straight ahead. Press your legs into the floor and flex your feet. Place your right hand palm-down on the floor alongside you to help keep your spine long and straight. Drop your shoulders down away from your ears. Stretch your left hand in front of you. Make a capital *L* with your pointer finger and thumb.

Move your L-shaped body to the left by rocking back and forth on your sit bones (your ischium). Steer by swiveling your L hand back and forth.

Move to the right and steer with your right hand, now that you know your left from right.

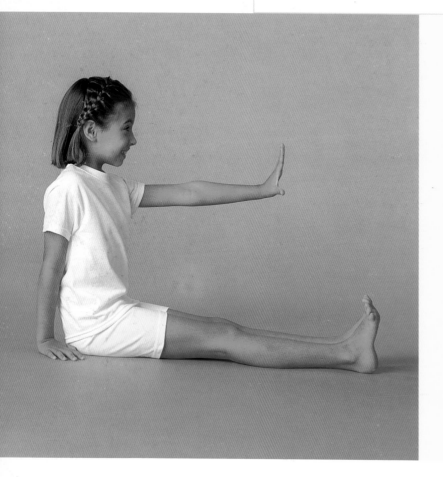

Elements

For young children, *L* is one of the letters that gets transposed. But usually around age five, most children can tell if the *L* is backward. Seeing the *L* shape of their hands and feeling the *L* shape of their body will help ingrain the letter *L*.

Laughing Language/Math Medley

ABCDEFGHIJK L MNOPQRSTUVWXYZ
What letters are to the left of the *L*?
What letters are to the right?
How many letters are on each side?

Draw a line from top to bottom down the middle of a sheet of paper. On the left side write *L* words that you know. On the right, write *R* words.

Musical Musings

Recite the alphabet in rhythm, with a breath or pause between each letter. If you're feeling really creative, rap the letters of the alphabet forward and backward.

Begin in Heel Sitting pose (page 20). Separate your knees a little bit and open your fingers to form lion claws. Place your claws on top of your thighs. Breathe in and puff up your proud lion chest with your breath. Open the back of your throat as you breathe out with a quiet, throaty "Rrrroar." Stretch your tongue out toward your chin. Quietly roar three times. Then get louder and do three more ripping roars. Growl, grunt, yawn, and purr, too.

Lions roar to protect their homes, attract mates, and scare away enemies. Powerful roars can be heard five miles away.

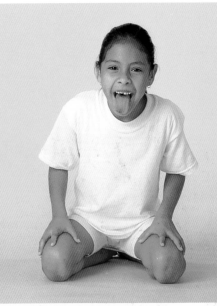

Elements

This pose opens the throat. It is especially helpful in winter months and for colds. It pulls up phlegm, which should be spit out to help clear the body of excess mucus. It can even help remedy bad breath.

Musical Musings/Ecological Echoes

Three different types of roars make up the lions' song:

> The prelude, or beginning, is generally soft, low moaning.
> The energy rises to a roar that generally goes from high to low, and ends with "Aaoouuu."
> The finale is staccato, with grunts that sound like "huh, huh, huh." (*Staccato* means "short and fast.")

Laughing Language

Lions have many different sounds in their language, and so do we:

A is for Aaoouuuu

G is for Grunt and Growl

H is for Huh

P is for Purr

R is for Roar

Y is for Yawn

Go through the alphabet and find a sound for each letter.

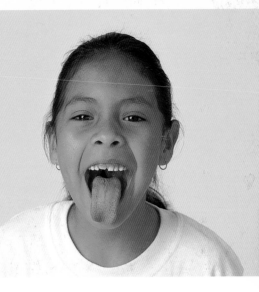

abcs

S Is for Snake

Slithering like a snake makes your spine feel fine.

Lie on your belly. Gently squeeze your legs together to shape your body long and strong, like a snake's. Place your hands under your shoulders and breathe in. Lift up your chest and head. Pull your shoulders down, away from your ears. Breathe out and hiss the *ssss* sound of the snake. Flick out your tongue. Lower your chest and rest on the ground. Repeat as many times as you like.

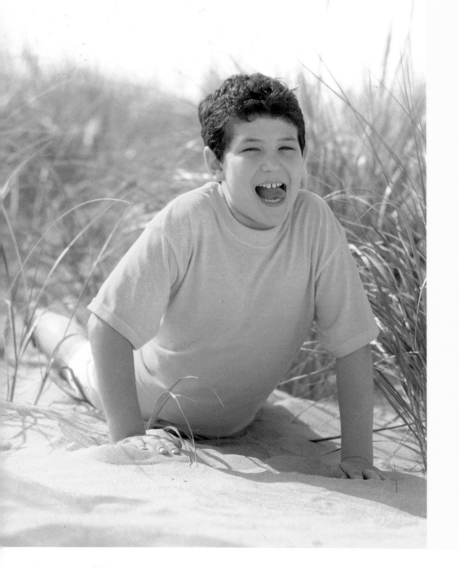

Elements

This pose is the favorite of many children, especially boys. Practicing the Snake will keep the spine and lower back flexible. This variation also exercises the tongue and opens the throat. When the snake is charmed, he is learning to follow nonverbal directions and enhance eye/brain/body coordination.

Put your infants or toddlers on your back while you practice this pose yourself. They'll enjoy the snake ride as you lift up and down and slither across the floor with them as your cargo. To finish up, coil around them and cuddle up.

Laughing Language

Make up "S" sentences, and put an "S" place in each. Here are some to get you started:

"Silly sloths scoot to Saturn."
"Super snails slide to Savannah."

Musical Musings

Play music from India to coax your snake's movements and broaden his musical tastes. Indian musicians play instruments with lovely names, like *sarangi, sitar, tabla, tambora,* and *tanpura*.

Snake Charmer

One person is the snake. The other is the snake charmer. The snake charmer squats in front of her snake and plays her flute. The snake pays close attention to his charmer: as she moves the flute, her snake follows it with his eyes and body: up and down, side to side, high and low. The snake charmer leads her snake in a winding dance.

The charmer guides her snake back down onto his belly, strokes him, and thanks him for a great job. She curls her snake into a ball and puts him back into the basket. Then they trade places for the next show.

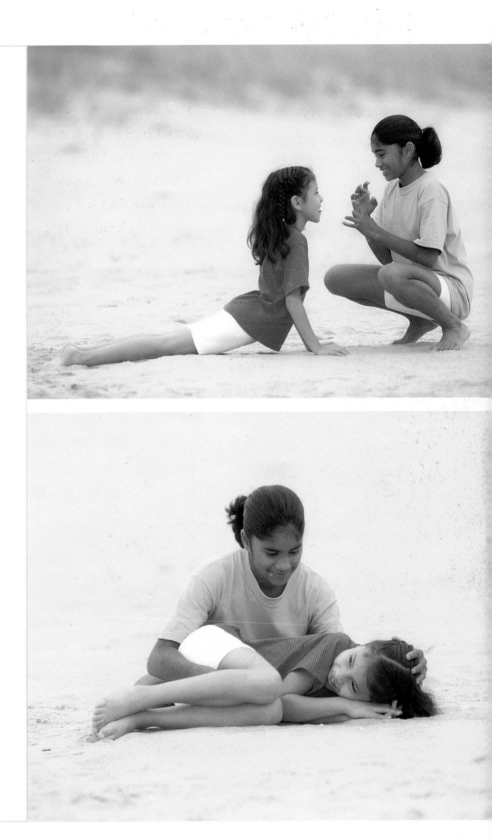

Ankle-Heel-Toe Walking

Your feet contain 52 bones, 66 joints, 38 muscles, and 214 ligaments. One quarter of all the bones in your body are in your feet.

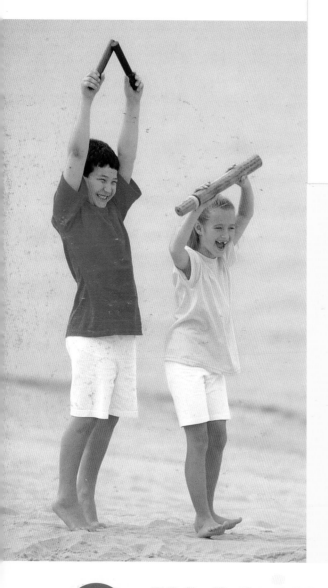

Put on your favorite music or make your own. Clap your hands to a beat or grab a pair of rhythm sticks.

Stand tall with your spine long. Lift your heels and walk high on your tiptoes. Then lower your heels to the floor, lift your toes in the air, and walk on your heels.

With feet flat on the floor, roll your ankles in toward each other. Balance on the inside edge of your feet (your arches) and walk around. Then roll your ankles away from each other, balance on the outside edge of your feet, and walk around.

This rhythmic walking on ankles, heels, and toes introduces you to all different parts of your feet. Can you feel them?

Elements

Try these four ways of walking in different combinations. Call out a direction and a speed—for example, "Heel walk real fast. Outer edges of the feet, nice and slow."

Invent different walking patterns, too—forward, backward, in a circle, zigzag, in a squat. Have him clap his hands or play his instrument in various positions—high, low, in behind or front.

Flexibility and muscle tone in the feet is an important part of overall fitness and can help prevent foot problems later in life.

The feet set the alignment of the body structure from the ground up. Good posture starts with happy feet.

Brain Balance

This pose takes coordination and communication between the body and the brain. Music is the right side of the brain. Following orders is the left side of the brain. This walking exercise keeps both sides of your brain running smoothly and communicating efficiently.

Awesome Anatomy/Visual Vignettes

Trace your feet and label the parts: toes, nails, heel, arch, ball. Add toe rings, tattoos, or nail polish to your drawings.

moving & grooving

Bug-Pickin' Chimp

Bend your knees and squat down on your feet. Walk around. Lead with your long arms and jump with your bent legs. On a soft surface, try "knuckle-walking."

Check your friends for bugs and nits. Pick some out and pretend to eat them.

Make monkey sounds. Roll back your lips and bare your teeth. Breathe with a "he-he-he" sound. Make puckered monkey lips and breathe with a "hoo-hoo-hoo" sound. Go back and forth.

You've cleaned each other up and fed yourselves, too. Good monkeys. Reward yourselves with a banana.

Monkeys love to "nit-pick." They search for bugs and insect eggs in each others' fur and eat them.

Elements

Bridge of Diamonds
Cooperation and taking care of one another is a good idea for all living things.

Math Medley
You picked ___ nits.
Your friend picked ____ nits.
How many nits did you pick together?

Musical Musings
Sing to the melody of "Five Little Monkeys."

"Bug-pickin' chimps went swinging
through the trees

They laughed and sang and breathed
"he-he."

Cleaned their fur till their coats
were nit-free

Then shared big bananas for all to see."

Ecological Echoes
Monkeys' arms are much longer than their legs. That's why they can swing through the trees, and knuckle-walk on the forest floor. Try it, and you'll wish you had monkey arms, too.

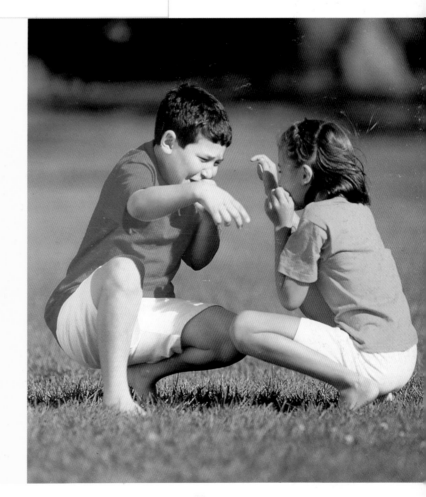

Roller Coaster

Roller coasters started as ice slides in seventeenth-century Russia. Sleds were rolled down steep slopes of wood covered with ice. One hundred years later the French added wheels and tracks.

1. Sit down with legs spread wide. Clasp your hands together around the waist of the person in front of you. As the roller coaster climbs up the hill, lean back.

2. Then lean forward as you speed downhill.

3. Be brave and raise your hands as you lean right and left. Screeeeeam. When you've had enough, stop the ride and collapse back. Rest.

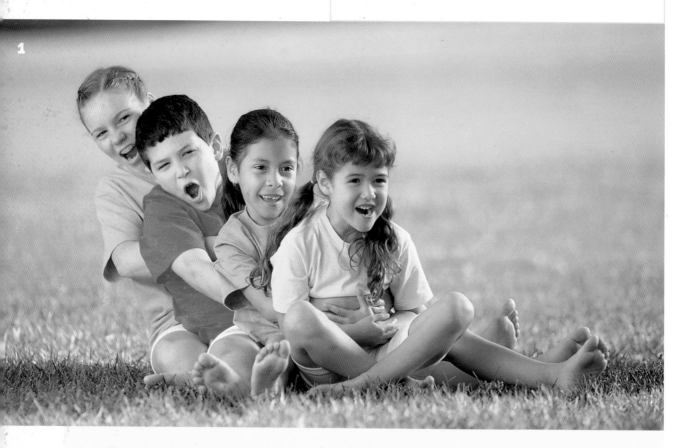

Elements

We All Win / Bridge of Diamonds
Take turns riding at the front of the roller coaster. Follow the leader. Move together as one. Enjoy the ride.

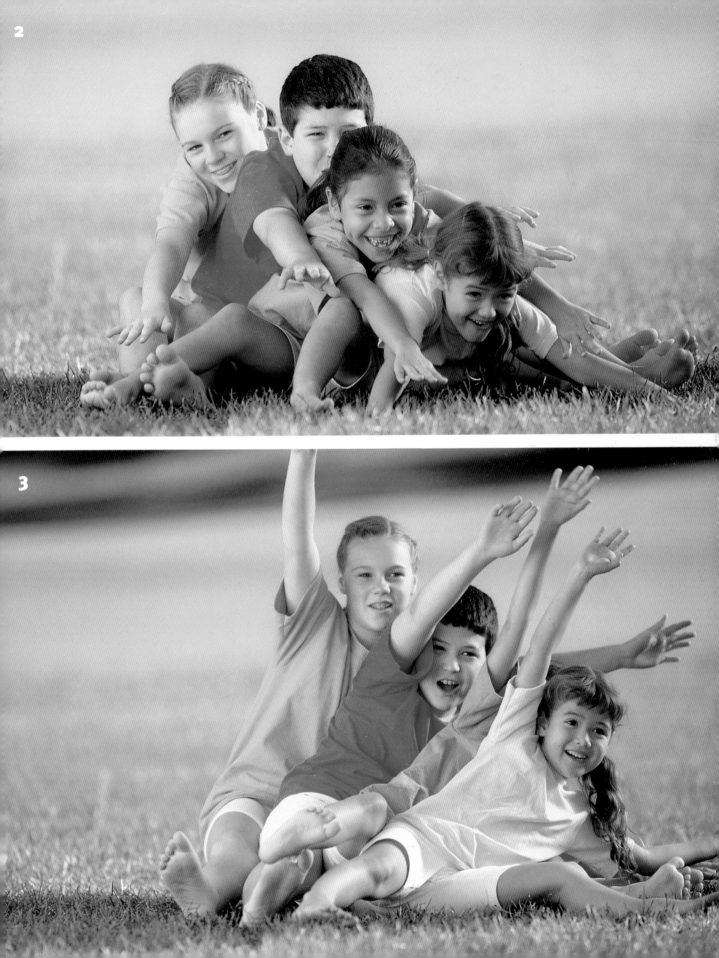

Spouting Dolphin

Dolphins, like whales, whistle through their blowholes to talk to each other.

Begin in All Fours pose (page 20). Lower your elbows to the floor. Make sure your knees are under your hips. Grasp your elbows with the opposite fingers to keep proper spacing. Try not to let your elbows spread wider than your shoulders.

Elements

Practicing Spouting Dolphin will build strength in the upper body, especially in the arms, shoulders, and back. Start with 3 rounds of Spouting Dolphin. When this becomes easy, increase by one round. Gradually build up by 3 at a time—6, 9, 12, and so on. This pose also strengthens the abdominal and leg muscles.

Ecological Echoes

Dolphins are mammals, like humans; they are not fishes. These mammals have lungs and breathe air through their blowholes at the top of their heads. When dolphins are underwater, they don't have to hold their breath, because they store oxygen in their blood and muscles, but they have to surface for a gulp of air every five minutes or so.

Musical Musings

By squeezing air back and forth between air sacs under their blowholes, they make clicking sounds to communicate. Create some dolphin melodies, using clicking sounds. Click away as you spout back and forth through the water.

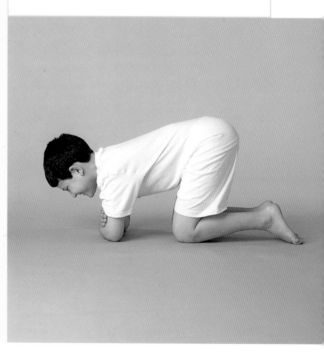

Move your lower arms forward, interlace your fingers, and make a triangle. Your hands are one point, and your elbows are the other two points. Breathe in and out, letting your spine lengthen and your tailbone lift up and back. Work your legs strongly. Press your heels to the floor.

Breathe out and in. Move your body forward so your chin touches down in front of your fingers. Then breathe out and lift out of the water.

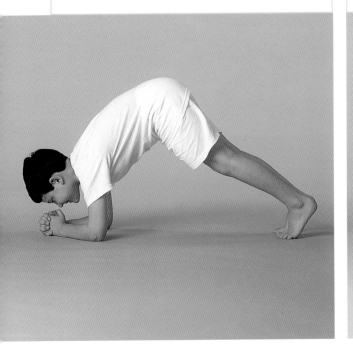

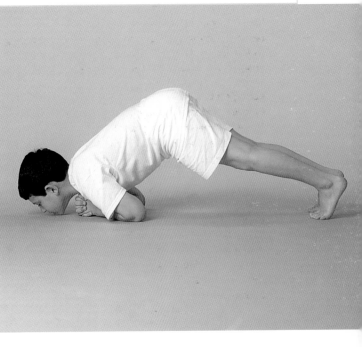

Row Your Boat

Rowing a boat takes strength and coordination. Your body works hard, yet the oars dip softly into the water without splashing too much.

Begin in L Sitting pose (page 20). Place both hands, palms down, alongside your hips. Lengthen your arms and spine. Lean back and lift your legs up. Balance on your sit bones (your ischium). Stretch your arms forward, palms facing each other. Breathe in and out. Practice 5 to 10 Dragon Breaths (page 28) in this position.

Row your arms forward. Sing "Row, Row, Row Your Boat." Reverse, and row your arms backward. Keep singing.

To rest in between repetitions, bring your legs down and fold forward into Peanut Butter & Jelly (pages 92–93). Then row forward and back two more times.

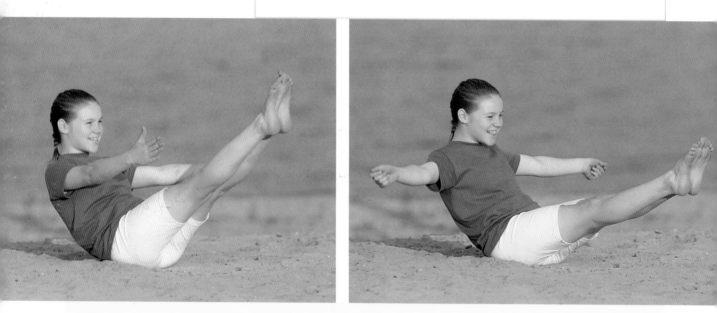

Elements
Over time, Row Your Boat will strengthen the stomach, back, and shoulder muscles, as well as tone the kidneys, liver, and intestines. When you sing and row, you can hold the pose longer.

Musical Musings
Sing "Row, Row, Row Your Boat." Do as many verses as you can while you practice the pose. If there are two or more rowers, sing the song in a round.

We All Win/Brain Balance
Practice Row Your Boat together. Sit side by side, hold hands, and balance. Row in unison. Synchronize your breath. Now row forward with your outer hands and row back with your holding hands; then reverse.

Polar Bear

When you feel a need to curl up or hibernate, try this pose.

Begin in Heel Sitting pose (page 20). Open your knees wide apart, toes touching behind you. Bend forward at the hips and slide your chest along the floor. Place your chin on the floor and put your paws over your nose to keep yourself warm. Breathe in and out.

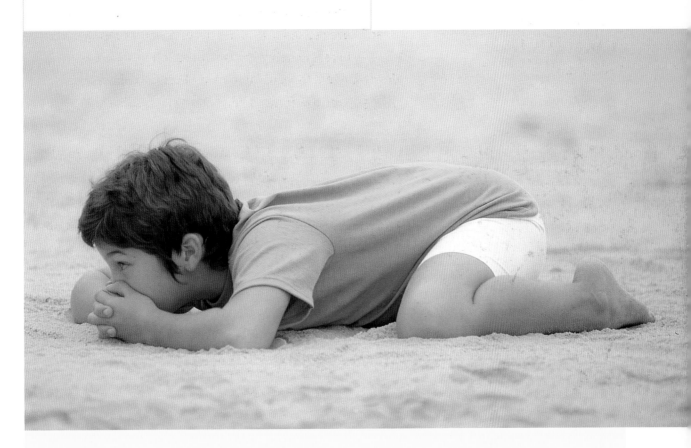

Elements
Lie in Polar Bear pose, facing your child. Gaze into her eyes. Mirror each other while practicing Eyes Around the Clock (pages 34–35). Then nuzzle your muzzles.

Bridge of Diamonds
Polar bears will frequently share a kill. They approach one another slowly, circle around the carcass, and then meekly offer a nose-to-nose greeting.

Visual Vignettes
An adult polar bear paw can measure 12 inches across. The claws are about 2 inches long. Use a compass and a ruler to draw a life-size bear paw. Color or paint it.

Math Medley
Polar bears have been known to swim 60 miles at one time, traveling about 6 miles an hour. That's a 10 hour swim! How far could they go in 5 hours?

Talking Turtle

Turtles travel light. Wherever they go, their homes go with them. Their shell is made of bone and is called a carapace. They wear it, sleep in it, live in it, and retreat into it.

1. Begin in L Sitting pose (page 20). Open your legs wide. Flex your feet. Lift your knees. Place your hands on the floor, inside your legs. Spread out your fingers.

2. Slide your hands and arms under your knees, as far away from each other as possible. Bend forward at the hips and lengthen your chest along the floor. Lift your head and look from side to side. Be a Talking Turtle. What will you say today?

3. Stretch your arms and legs as far out as you can. Lengthen your upper body on the floor. Tuck in your chin. Now you have retreated into your shell. Pull all of your senses inward and rest. Stay in your shell for 10 seconds. Breathe in, lift your head and talk. Breathe out, tuck your chin in, retreat, and be quiet. Come in and out of your shell a few times.

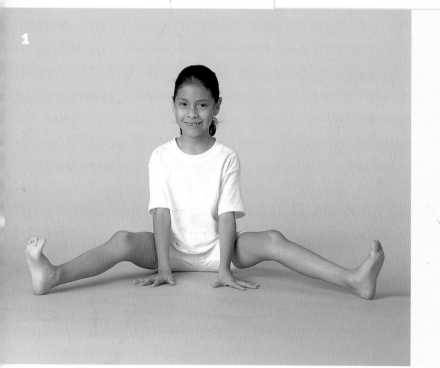

Elements

Talking Turtle juxtaposes the outward, talkative nature of a child with the ability to withdraw and be quiet. Physically, the pose tones the spine, activates the organs, and stretches the groin and legs.

Laughing Language

Sit across from one another in Talking Turtle. Take turns coming in and out of your shell as you ask and answer questions. The first turtle speaks, with her head up. The second turtle listens, with his head down. Then switch roles.

Ecological Echoes

Turtles have nostrils at the top of their heads so they can breathe while most of their body is under water.

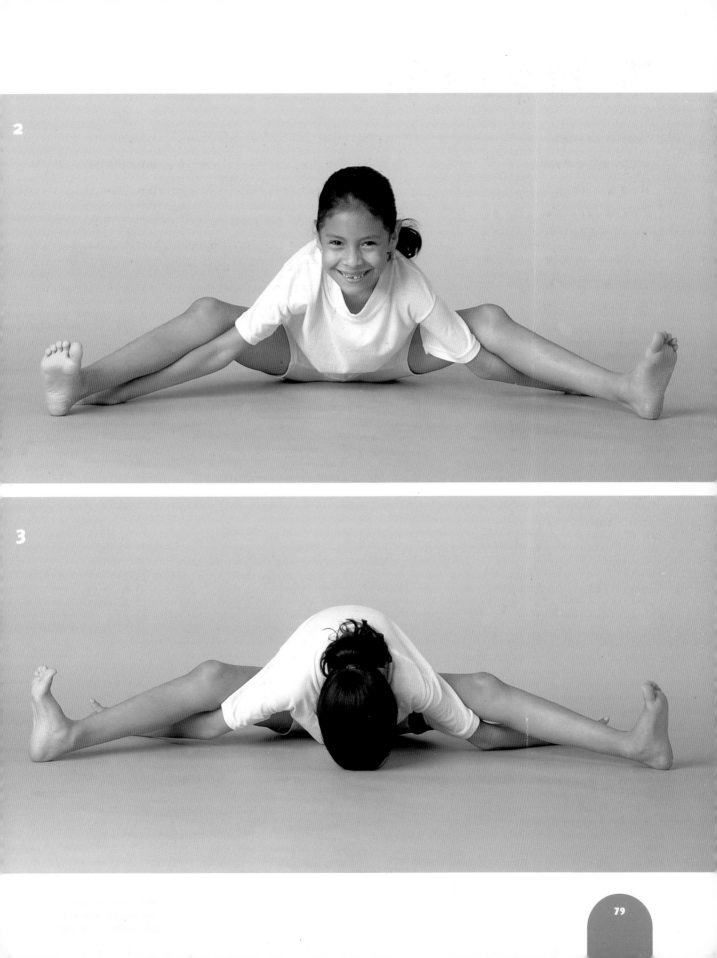

Bubble Fish

If you were a fish, you might live in a salty ocean, a raging river, a quiet pond, or maybe an aquarium in your best friend's room.

Lie on your back, arms at your sides. Bring the bottoms of your feet together and open your knees outward to make a fish tail. Press your feet together and flap your legs up and down. Slide your hands, palms down, underneath your backside. Squeeze your shoulders together, press into your elbows and lower arms, and arch your back as your chest lifts off the floor. Place the top of your head on the floor.

Imagine you have gills instead of lungs. Fish breathe by taking water in through their mouths and pushing it out through their gills. Feel your gills open and close as you breathe. Make fish lips and blow bubbles.

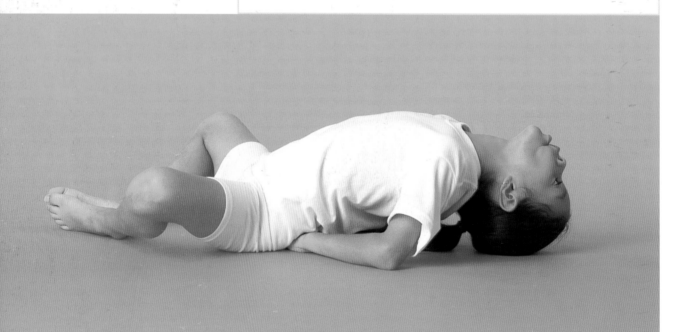

Elements
This is a wonderful pose to aid the endocrine system; it also opens the chest and breaks up tension in the back.

Brain Balance
With the head upside down, the flow of blood and oxygen to the brain increase, making this pose simultaneously energizing and calming.

Musical Musings
Recordings of watery sound effects are calming to the mind, and put the body in a flowing and fluid mood.

Swan

Begin in All Fours pose (page 20). Bend your lower legs, pointing your toes to the sky, and glide your body forward. Lift your chest and lengthen your graceful neck. You are a swan, sailing from side to side as you move smoothly through the water. Breathe in and out.

A vinyasa is a flow of poses linked together through breath and movement. Begin as one animal . . . breathe. . . . turn into another one . . . breathe.

Elements

Help your child repeat the Transformer series using the opposite leg. Encourage her to invent her own *vinyasas*. Play Transformers using other poses in this book, and then use your imagination. There's no limit to the combinations you can put together.

Laughing Language/ Visual Vignettes

Write down the Transformer series you create. Draw them too. Share your series with others on the YogaKids® Web site (see page 124 for address).

Math Medley

How many different poses are in your own Transformers series? How many times do you repeat each pose? Count them.

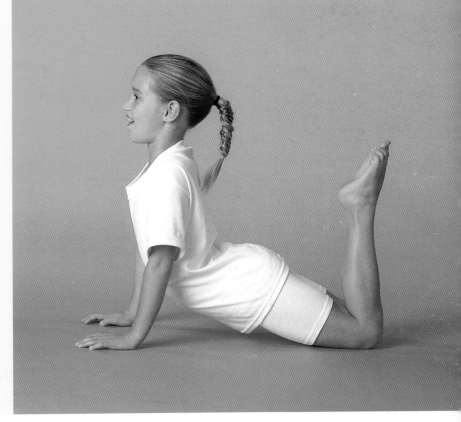

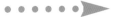

pattern & rhythm

Down Diggety Doggy Down

Lower your legs, bend your toes forward, and pull your heels down as you push up so your legs straighten. Lengthen your arms and spine and lift your hips. You are a dog, barking, growling, marking your territory.

Lunge

Now sit up and beg: Step the right foot forward into a lunge and place your hands flat on either side of that foot.

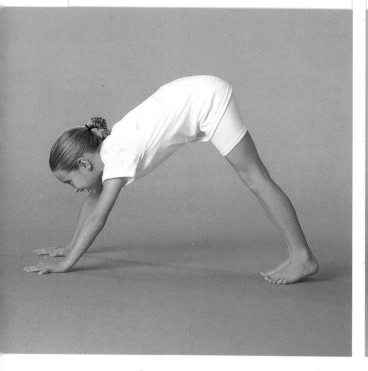

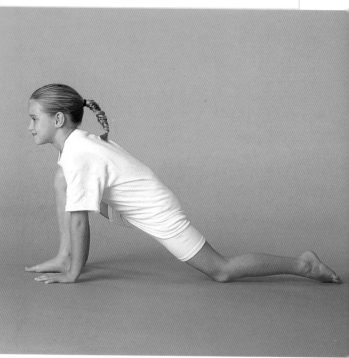

pattern & rhythm

Lift your hands onto the upper thigh, above the knee. Breathe in—lift your chest. Breathe out—move your lower body toward the floor.

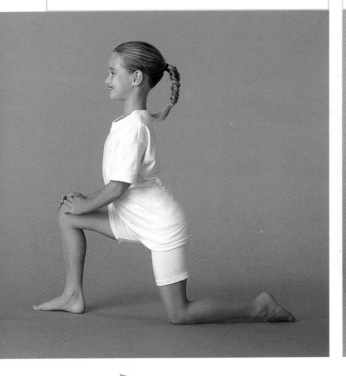

Then place your hands back down on the floor. . .

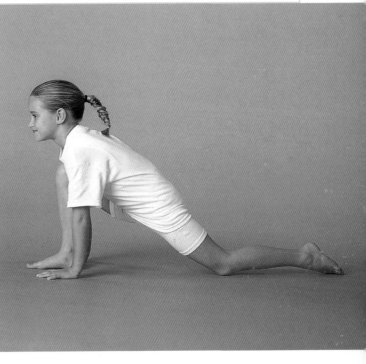

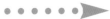

Snake

Keeping your arms straight, lower your hips to the floor. Breathe in: lift your chest forward. Breathe out: your legs and toes trail behind as you transform into a snake. Hiss and sway.

. . . and bend your left toes forward, stepping your right leg back. Transform again to Down Diggety Doggy Down.

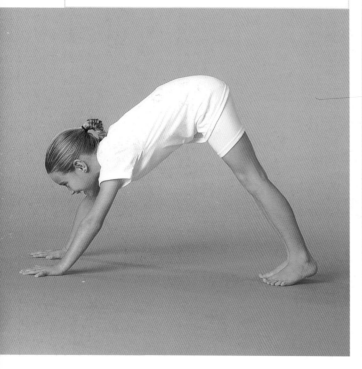

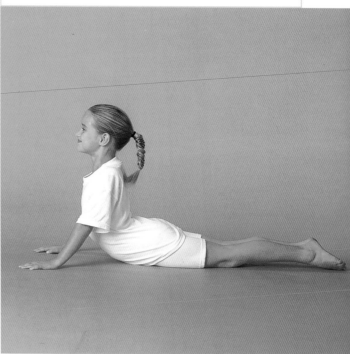

Extended Child's Pose

Press through your hands and push back with your backside until you are sitting on your heels. Stretch your arms out in front of you, palms on the floor. Rest your head. Breathe in and out. Now you are another kind of animal—a human child.

Polar Bear

Open your knees and bring your hands to your face. Gently cup your hands over your nose. Breathe in and out. Close your eyes and feel your breath warming your nose. You are a polar bear.

Start over again as a Swan. Try to do 5 to 10 rounds of Transformers.

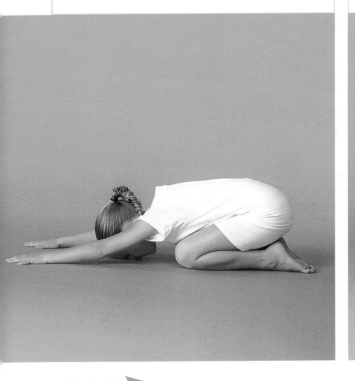

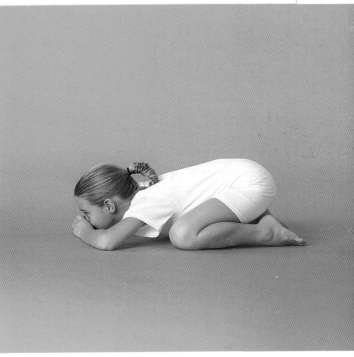

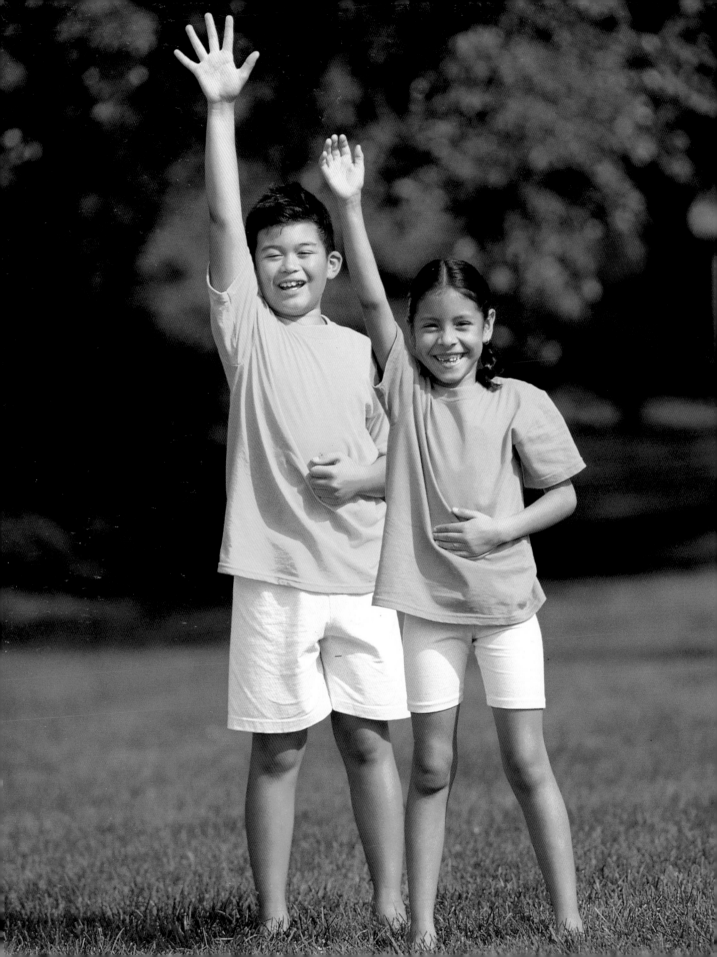

Begin in Open Mountain pose (page 49).
Breathe in and reach up
high with an outstretched hand. Grab a
piece of sunshine and pull the power
into your solar plexus—your inner sun.
Exhale with a "Hah" breath.
Repeat with the other arm. Alternately
reach with the left and right arms.
As you practice, increase the force of
your breath. Can you work up to 2
minutes? Feel the power of the sun
shining inside you.

**Pull the power of the sun
from the sky to fuel
your dreams. Feel your
belly smile and shine.**

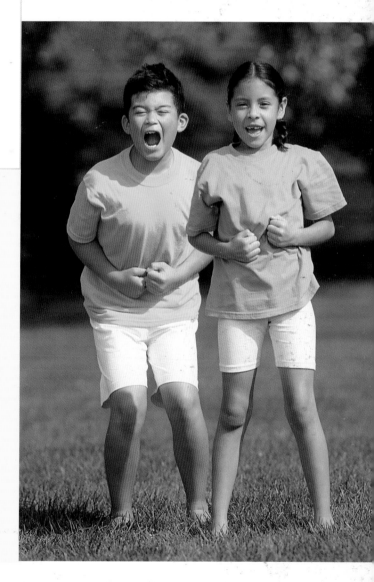

Elements

The solar plexus is located between the chest and
the navel. It is the third chakra (see page 106), the
place of personal power. The Japanese call it the
hara. If your child practices any of the martial arts,
he might be familiar with this concept. If he's feeling
fearful or needs a boost of confidence, suggest
practicing this pose with an affirmation:

I share my power in peaceful ways.
When I feel insecure, I reach for the sun.
When I feel afraid, I turn on the light inside of me.

(See page 111 for affirmations to try with this pose.)

Musical Musings

See page 117 for the YogaKids® song that was
written for this pose.

Bridge of Diamonds

Children can learn to understand and trust their
own power. We do not need to exert force over
anyone or anything. We can live in balance together.

Om a Little Teapot Triangle

This is our version of the classic asana called *trikonasana,* **the Triangle pose (***tri*** means "three,"** *kona* **means "angle," and** *asana* **means "pose"). Three angles form a triangle. Can you find the triangles in this pose?**

Elements

This pose increases strength and flexibility of the feet, legs, hips and neck. It helps lengthen the spine, too.

With young children, ignore the detailed directions of the feet. For children approximately 10 and older, or if they have been practicing for a while, we can begin to give them more details on structure and alignment.

Bridge of Diamonds
Instead of beginning this classic teapot rhyme with *I'm,* we start with *Om.* The yogis say that Om is the sound of the universe. (See page 109 for *Om.*)

Math Medley
There are three different types of triangles:

Equilateral (all sides are equal)

Isosceles (two sides are equal)

Scalene (all sides are unequal)

See how many different triangles you can make with your legs and arms.

Begin in Mountain pose (page 49). Jump your feet and arms apart.

1. Turn your right foot so it points to the right. Turn your left toes as far to the right as you can. Imagine a line from the back of your right heel straight into the middle of your left arch. Line up your feet on this imaginary line, to provide an even base for your triangle pose.

Press down evenly through both feet and feel strength in your legs. Place your left hand on your hip as the teapot handle. Bend your right arm to form the spout.

Sing the "I'm a Little Teapot" song, with these variations:

Om a little teapot short and stout.
Here is my handle.
Here is my spout.

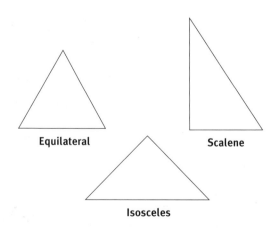

Equilateral   Scalene

Isosceles

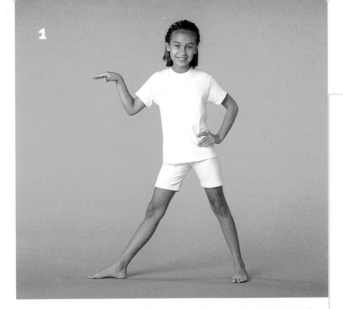

1

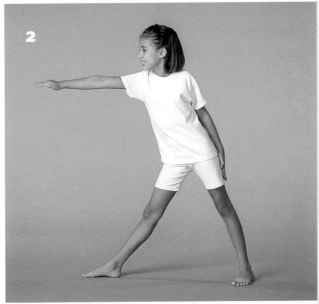

2

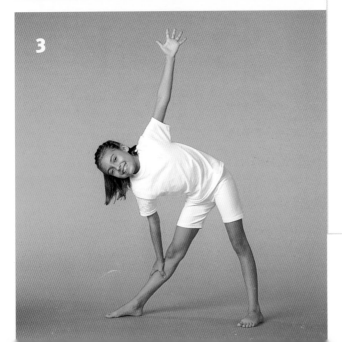

3

2. Release your left hand from your hip and slide it down your leg. Stretch your right arm straight out to the side, lengthen your right ribcage, and move your hips left.

> *When I get all steamed up,*
> *I reach out.*

3. Tilt your upper body to the right, your hips shift more to the left. Drop your right hand to your right leg. Raise your left arm.

> *Then tip me over and*
> *pour me up.*

If you feel yourself pitched too far forward, lift your right hand higher on the leg and rotate your chest skyward.

If it's comfortable, turn your head and look up. If not, look forward or down.

Wiggle your fingers and straighten up with your arms still extended out to the sides. Jump back to center. Turn your feet to the left. Repeat on the opposite side.

Rocking Horse

In adult yoga, this pose is called the Bow. But we like to move forward and back like a rocking horse. Get ready to rock!

Lie on your belly. Bend your knees and reach back to take hold of your ankles one at a time. Lift and broaden your chest as you squeeze your shoulder blades and inner thighs together. Look forward and bring your feet toward the sky. Notice how the entire back of your body contracts, so that the front of your body can open and lift like a proud horse. Take strong breaths in and out, as you begin to rock. Increase your rocking time with regular practice.

Do three rocking horses. Rest in the Child's Pose (page 33 and 85), full or extended, when you get tired.

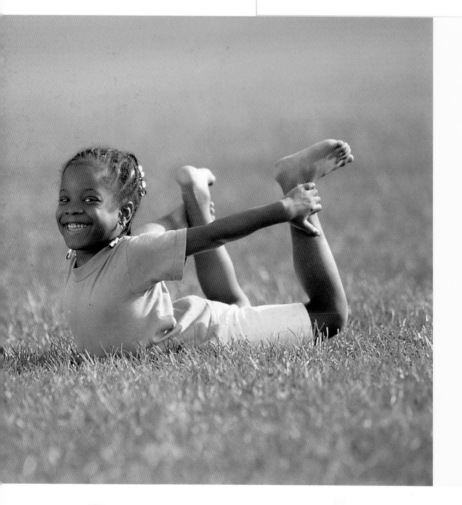

Elements

This backbend strengthens the spine as well as the shoulders and legs. It stimulates the kidneys and adrenal glands, too. The rocking motion massages the digestive organs.

Rocking Horse is an excellent way to feel the *prana* (energy, life force) of the breath enlivening the body. The more *prana* you can generate, the longer you'll be able to rock.

Backbends and forward bends have opposite effects. Backbends energize; forward bends calm.

Musical Musings

Sing "The Rocking Horse Song" (page 113) or any rhythmic, rocking song you like.

Visual Vignettes

Close your eyes and imagine an adventure on horseback. Where will you travel together? What will you see? Draw a picture of it.

Wheel

Children of all ages love to practice the Wheel. Moving into this pose can give you instant energy.

Lie on your back. Bend your knees and place your feet flat on the floor, heels in close to your backside. Raise your arms up over your head and bend your elbows. Place your palms flat on the floor beside your ears with the fingertips pointing toward your shoulders. Pull your elbows toward each other. Press down into your hands and feet, as your straighten your arms and legs, and your chest and thighs lift toward the sky.

Imagine a wheel underneath you, supporting the curve of your spine in this convex shape.

Elements

Help your child maintain proper alignment in this pose. Support her back with your hands, lifting her spine into her body, as her rib cage expands.

With regular and attentive practice, tremendous strength and flexibility of the spine and whole body will develop. Wheel opens the heart chakra (see page 106 for more on chakras).

Dromedary Delight (pages 42–43) is a good preparation for Wheel.

Affirmations

Try making some "affirmations" — statements about yourself that make you feel good. Use the affirmations on page 111, or make up your own.

Brain Balance

Whenever the head is lower than the heart, blood flow to the brain is increased. Wheel oxygenates the brain and awakens the mind.

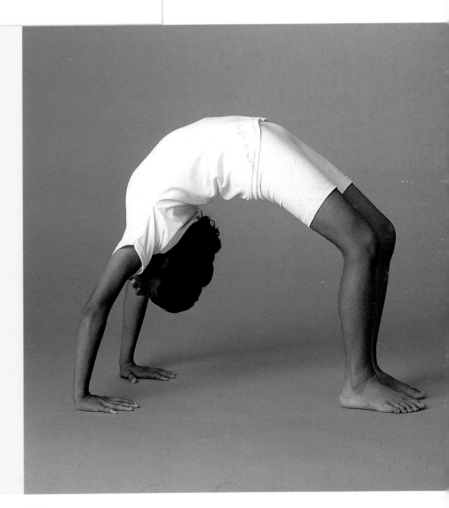

Peanut Butter & Jelly

The sweetness of jelly and the saltiness of peanut butter make a great combination. The average child eats 1,500 PB&J sandwiches before she graduates from high school. How many do you think you've eaten so far?

Elements

PB&J stretches and lengthens the hamstrings and the entire back of the body from head to toe. It tones the liver and kidneys, improves circulation, releases tension, and soothes the nervous system.

Awesome Anatomy

Together with your child, say each body part out loud as he spreads the peanut butter and jelly: "Peanut butter feet, peanut butter ankles, peanut butter shins, jelly thighs, jelly belly . . ." Help him substitute the names of muscles and bones (see anatomy charts on page 104–105).

Laughing Language

Add all kinds of real and outrageous ingredients: bananas, sprinkles, dinosaur tails, pizza . . . yucky or delicious, encourage kids to use their imaginations. Write down their PB&J recipes. Make up a menu for a PB&J restaurant.

Begin in L Sitting pose (page 20).

1. Reach up and grab the peanut butter and jelly jars that have magically appeared in the air.

2. Rub PB&J all over your hands and smear it between your toes.

3. Spread PB&J on your legs and on your belly.

4. Wash your face and hair in peanut butter and jelly.

Stretch your arms up again, fold forward at the hip hinge, and lengthen your spine and upper body over your lower body to make a peanut-butter-and-jelly sandwich. Press the backs of your legs into the floor. Press your chest into your legs. Squish those two pieces of bread together. Can you reach your toes to wash them clean?

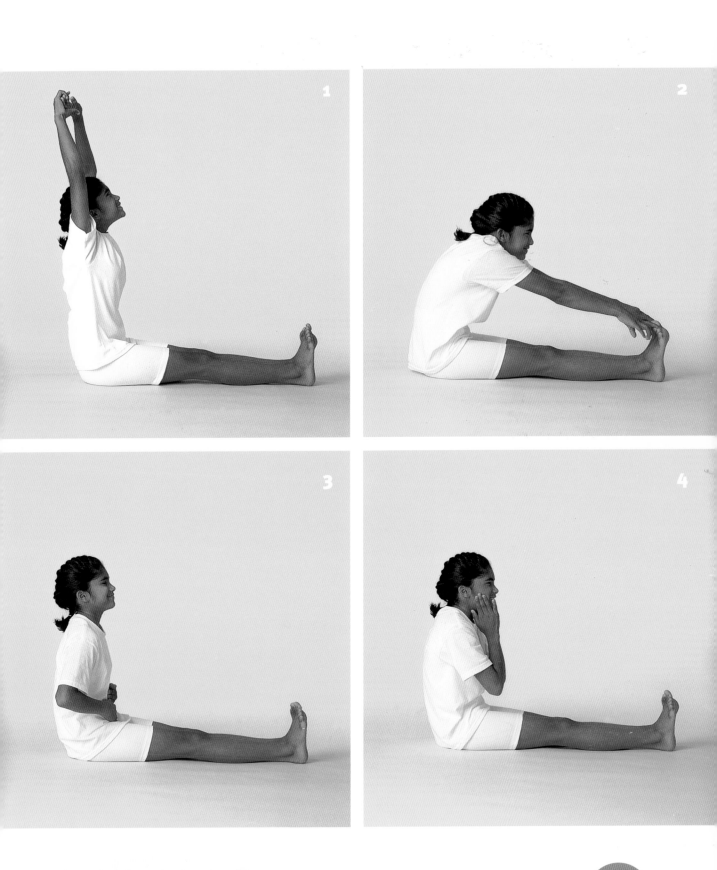

Swinging Pretzel

According to legend, an Italian monk invented the pretzel almost 1,400 years ago from the way children folded their arms in prayer.

1. Sit cross-legged. Take hold of your left ankle and foot and place them high up on your right thigh. Now you are in the half-pretzel. If you can, do the same thing with the other ankle. When both ankles are on both thighs, you're in the full pretzel. Switch legs so that each gets a turn on top.

2. Now swing your pretzel: Spread your fingers and palms flat on the floor just behind your knees. Press them down as you lengthen your arms. Lift your bottom and legs up off the floor. With strong arms and breathing, swing your pretzel back and forth.

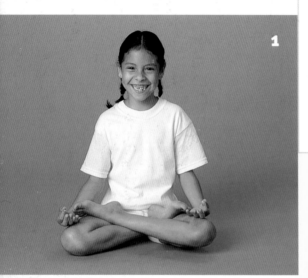

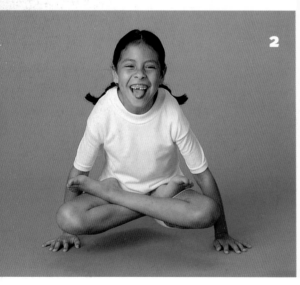

Elements
In adult yoga, this pose is known as half lotus or full lotus. The pretzel develops strength and flexibility in the knee, hip, and ankle joints. Child's Pose, Bow and Arrow, Talking Turtle, and 360-Degree Owl also build flexibility in the hips.

Laughing Language
The word *pretzel* is derived from two other languages. The word for pretzel comes from the Latin *pretiole*, "little gift." The Italian word is *bracciatelli*, "small arms."

Awesome Anatomy
Girls generally have an easier time sitting pretzel-style because a girl's pelvis is thin and wide. A boy's smaller and thicker pelvis makes it more difficult for boys to pretzel their legs.

Musical Musings/Brain Balance
If you like mustard on your pretzel, pretend to squirt some on your legs with your imaginary mustard jar. Go back and forth, covering your legs with mustard and chanting "crisscross with mustard sauce." Do three rounds in both directions. If you are a lefty, use your right hand. If you are a righty, use your left. Your brain is "grooving" a new pattern to link both sides together.

Birthday Candle Series

Rock 'n' Roll

Sit cross-legged. Take hold of your toes from the outer side of your knees. Breathe in and lift up your chest. Breathe out and tuck in your chin.

Elements

Encourage your child to sing "Happy Birthday," while in the candle pose. It will increase the length of time she stays in the pose. The poses in the series can also be practiced individually. Remember to let your breath flow in and out throughout this series.

When your child is in Birthday Candle, gently lift her legs to help her get more of her weight onto her shoulders. Shoulder stands are considered the best of all asanas, because of their enormous benefits, especially to the endocrine system.

Brain Balance

Whenever we cross the midline of the body in our movements, we stimulate much greater communication between the left and right sides of the brain. But for some children, crossing the legs but not the arms in Rock 'n' Roll can be very challenging. The alternative is to not cross the legs at all: bend the knees and grab the big toes with the hands of the same side. Then roll forward and back.

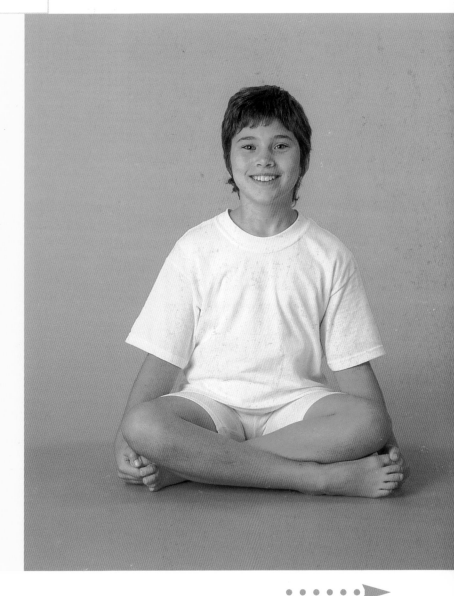

upside down

Breathe in and out. Round your back and roll backward. Extend your crossed legs over your head. Roll forward, tuck your legs, and sit up again. Do this 2 to 3 times to loosen up your spine, back, and legs. Re-cross your legs the other way, then roll another 2 to 3 times.

Plough

Breathe in and out. Roll backward in Rock 'n' Roll. Let go of your toes, bend your elbows, and use your hands to support and lift your back. Straighten your legs and lift them past your head until your bent toes touch the floor. Squeeze your shoulders and elbows together. Breathe in and out for 30 to 60 seconds. To relax in this pose, bend the knees and rest them on the floor on either side of the head. Rest your hands at the back of your knees.

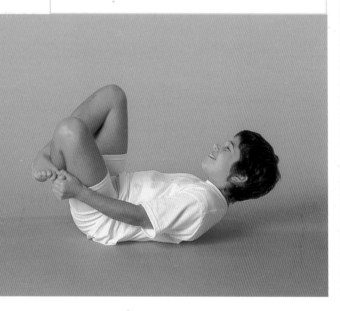

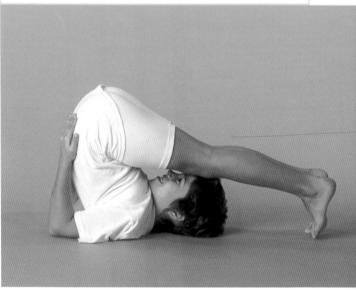

upside down

Birthday Candle

Continue to let your breath flow in and out. From Plough, lift the legs straight up to the ceiling. Rest your weight on your shoulder blades. Lift your chest. Your feet are the candle flames—have someone light the candle, or blow with enough power to ignite the flame yourself. Wiggle your toes to make the flames flicker. Tuck your chin to keep your neck relaxed. Sing "Happy Birthday." Take a big breath in and blow out your candle.

Bridge

From Birthday Candle, bend one knee at a time and drop that leg down to the floor in front of you. Follow with the other leg. Place the feet hip-width apart and press them into the floor. Walk the elbows closer in toward one another. Place your hands however it's comfortable to support your lower back and pelvis. Lift your chest and arch your spine. Gradually build up your strength until you can stay in Bridge for 10 breaths in and 10 breaths out. To come out of the pose, lift up your heels, place your hands flat on the floor, and roll the spine down, vertebra by vertebra, from top to bottom. To complete this series, come into Bubble Fish (page 80).

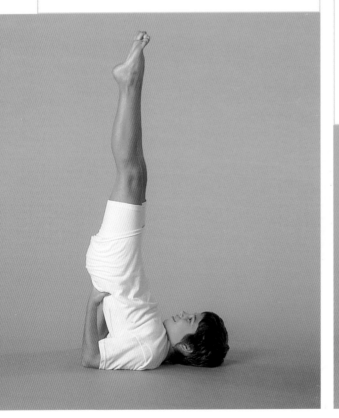

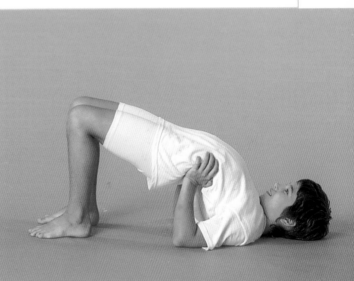

upside down

Handstand

A handstand is just an upside-down Mountain pose. The hands are where the feet are, and the feet are where the head is.

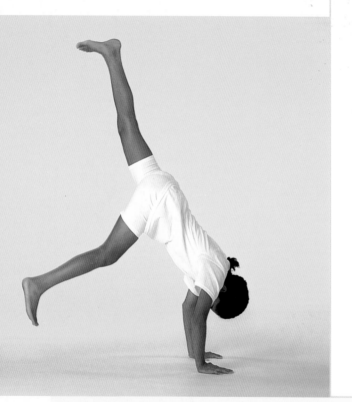

You'll need a wall nearby when you do this pose. Begin in Down Diggety Doggy Down (pages 40–41) with your back to the wall. Place your hands, with fingers fanned outward, shoulder-width apart, a few inches from the wall. Rise up on your toes and tiptoe toward your hands until your shoulders are right over your wrists.

Practice kicking up one leg at a time with pendulum kicks (legs as long and straight as possible). Rest your heels on the wall—first one, then both—so your body will "feel" the correct placement. With pendulum legs, practice, and confidence, you will stand on your hands.

Look down toward the floor behind you. Push the floor away with your hands and strong arms. Gently squeeze your feet and legs together as they stretch skyward. To come out of the pose, bring one leg at a time back down to the floor. Rest in Child's Pose (page 33) or Ragdoll (page 45).

Elements

Always "spot" your child in this pose; stand at her side and be ready to assist. As her pendulum kicks get closer to the wall, guide her legs upward and help her get into the handstand. Follow the alignment instructions above.

This pose is about overcoming fear. Try not to let fear get in your way. Encourage your child to practice safely and accurately. Most children love this pose: our responsibility is to make sure they do it properly.

Insist on pendulum kicks. Donkey kicks are kicks with bent legs. They are fun, but it will be almost impossible to get up with donkey kicks.

Visual Vignettes

If you are afraid to try this pose, draw a picture of yourself in this position to build your confidence. You'll be able to see yourself already doing it. Draw it. See it. Do it. Try some affirmations, too. "I am tall and proud, upside down with my hands on the ground." Or keep telling yourself, "I can do it. I can do it. I can do it."

upside down

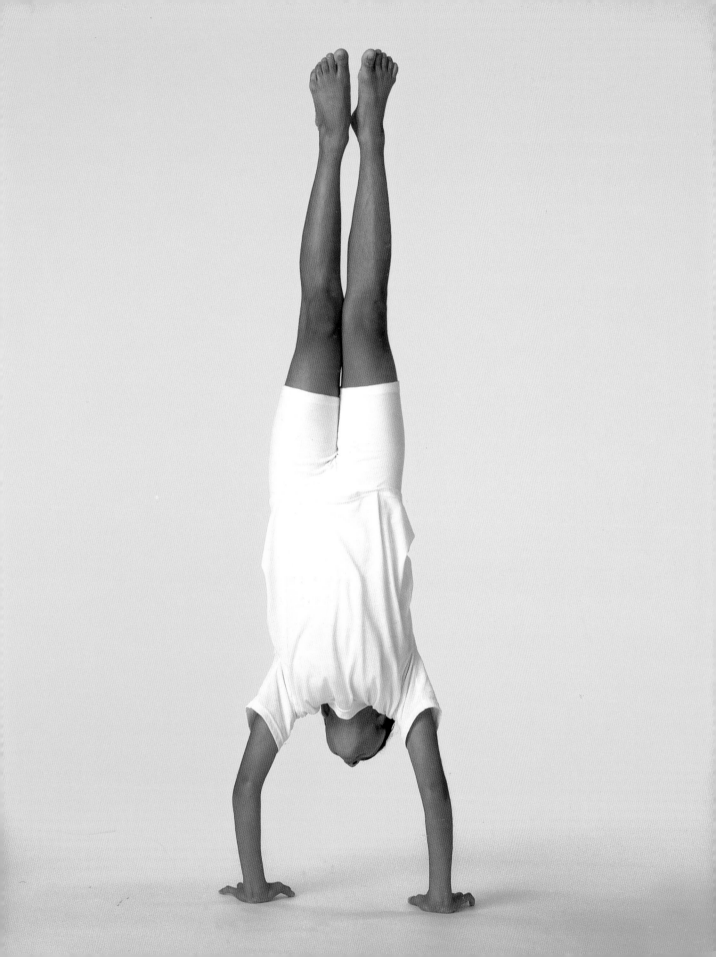

Lemon Toes

In Sanskrit, the ancient language of yoga, this pose is called *savasana*, from *sava*, "dead body"; we know it as the Corpse pose. Despite its name, it has many benefits. Lying perfectly still calms, balances, and renews.

Elements

Children enjoy herbal eye pillows or an animal friend on their bellies (see page 12). They love having their feet rubbed with peppermint- or lavender-scented lotions. They might like to be covered in a soft blanket, too.

Even though this pose looks simple, it is difficult to lie still. Remember how babies are swaddled? If your child is having trouble lying quiet, try some of these techniques:

The Enchilada: Roll her up, or let her roll herself in a yoga mat or blanket.

Count Dracula: Fold a large blanket into a triangle. Wrap him up like Dracula lying in his coffin, his head at the point of the blanket.

Some children feel afraid and defenseless lying on their backs. If the only way they can be still is to lie on their stomachs or sides, let them begin there. In time, they will become more comfortable and feel less vulnerable.

Turn the lights low.

Quiet Quests

Guide your child with visualizations like the Magical Cloud Carpet Ride (page 108).

Musical Musings

Introduce different types of music during the relaxation time. See page 117 for suggestions.

1. Lie on your back. Imagine that your toes are straws, sipping sour lemonade up from the bottom to every part of your body. Hold your breath as your toes curl and pucker. Breathe out as you relax your toes. Work your way up your legs, belly, chest, and arms, sipping, puckering, breathing, and relaxing.

Make a sourpuss face. Tighten up your nose, eyes, cheeks, teeth, and forehead. Let your hair curl. Hold it, squeeze it, tense it. Release. Finally, tighten your whole body at once. Hold it for 5 to 10 seconds. Completely release. Relax. Feel the difference between sour, tight, and tense, and the sweetness of relaxation.

2. Now you're ready for *savasana*. Your body relaxes into the floor. Your quiet breathing soothes your nervous system as your belly and chest gently move. Clear your mind of all thoughts. Stay in *savasana* for at least a minute, gradually building up to 10 to 15 minutes. Stay awake but totally relaxed and peaceful— sleeping is not *savasana*.

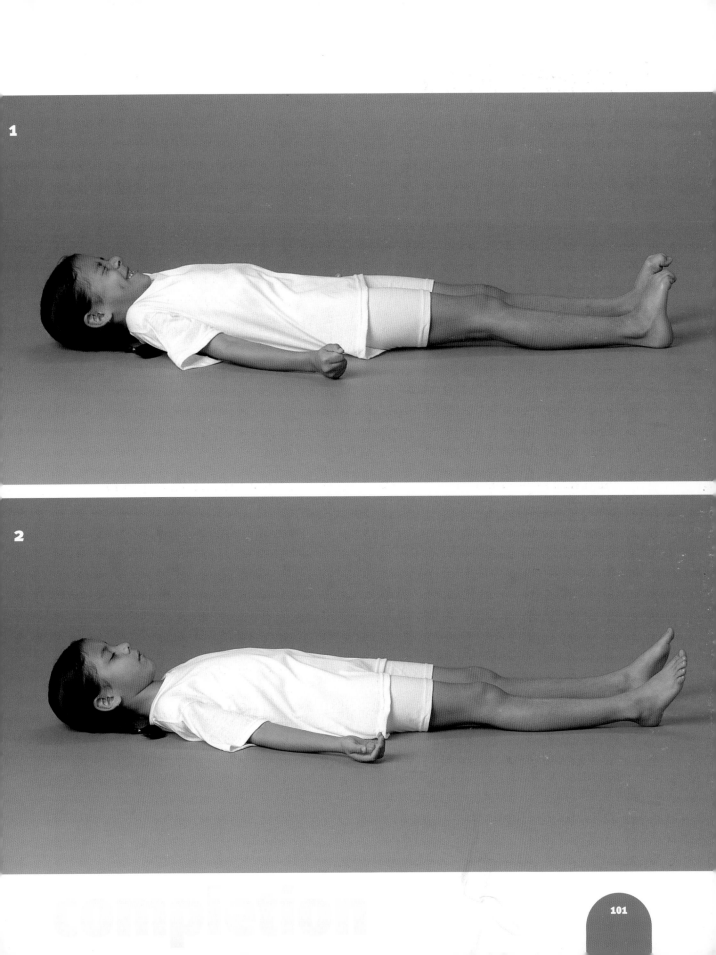

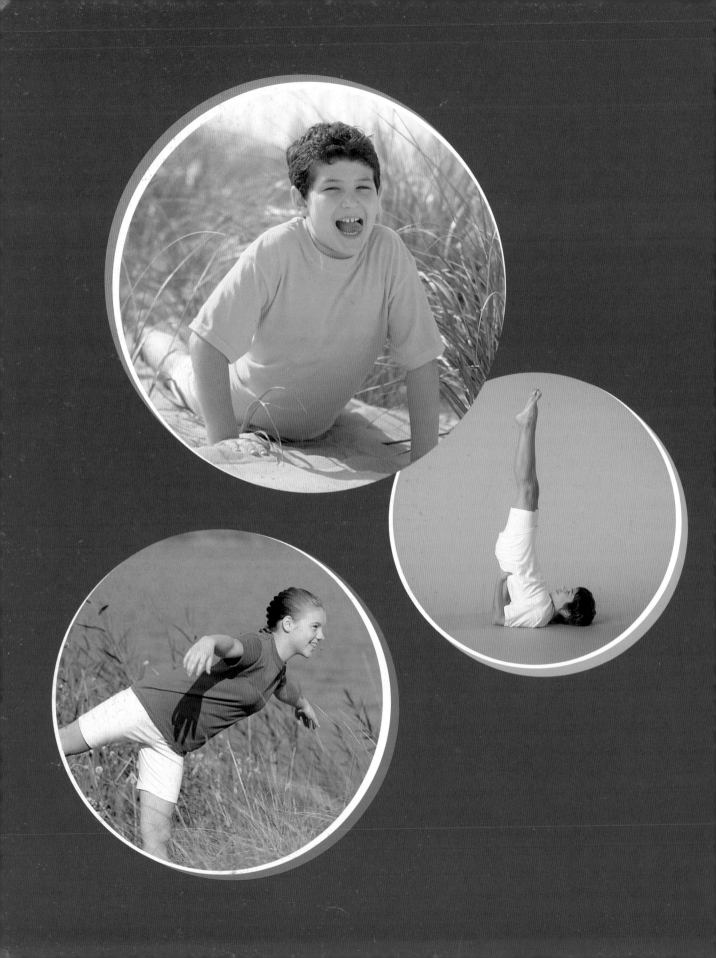

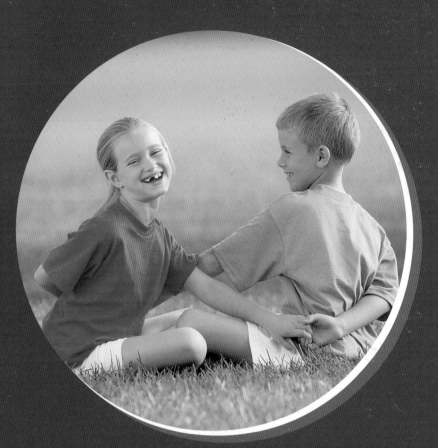

elements & more

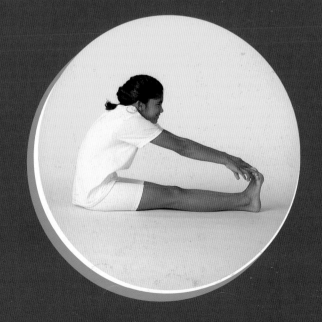

Awesome Anatomy

Awesome Anatomy is a way to help your child become aware of her own body. Once the deltoid has a name, she'll be more aware of it, and she'll know how to exercise it and what it does. Likewise, when she knows where her vertebrae are, she'll feel them stack neatly as she stands straight and tall in Mountain or sits upright in L Is for Left. Children love learning about themselves, and this is a great place to start.

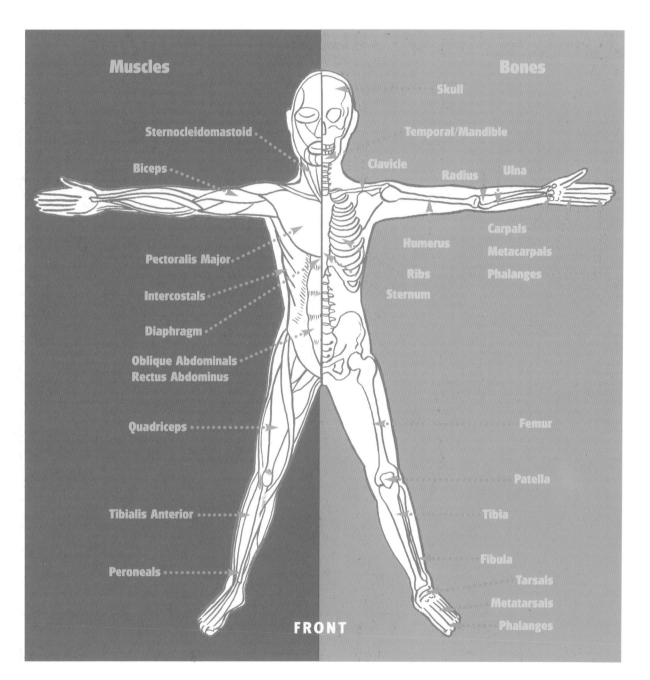

Muscles

- Sternocleidomastoid
- Biceps
- Pectoralis Major
- Intercostals
- Diaphragm
- Oblique Abdominals
- Rectus Abdominus
- Quadriceps
- Tibialis Anterior
- Peroneals

Bones

- Skull
- Temporal/Mandible
- Clavicle
- Radius
- Ulna
- Humerus
- Carpals
- Metacarpals
- Ribs
- Phalanges
- Sternum
- Femur
- Patella
- Tibia
- Fibula
- Tarsals
- Metatarsals
- Phalanges

FRONT

Like other elements, Awesome Anatomy grows with the children. Very young kids are probably just learning names for their body parts and where their internal organs are, so I recommend using the common names: when they show an interest in it, or when you feel they're ready, introduce a few scientific names. Use these diagrams as a starting point, along with the anatomy books listed on page 122.

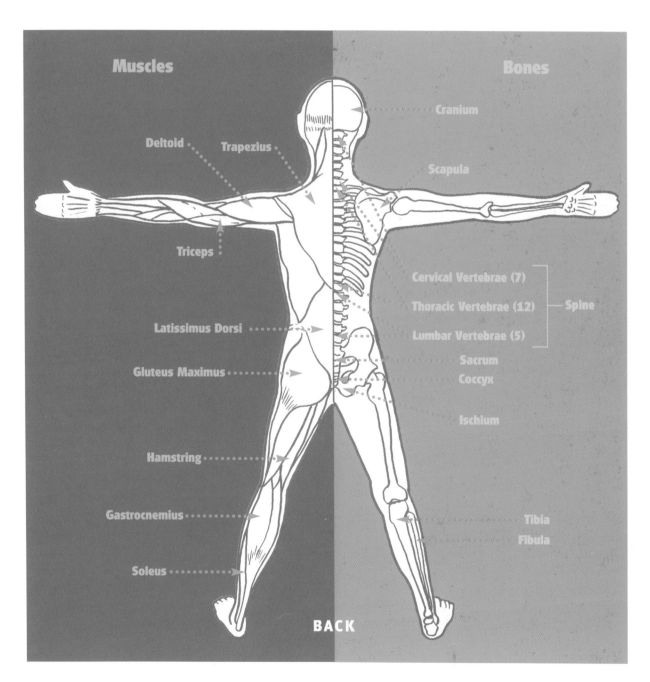

Muscles

Deltoid
Trapezius
Triceps
Latissimus Dorsi
Gluteus Maximus
Hamstring
Gastrocnemius
Soleus

Bones

Cranium
Scapula
Cervical Vertebrae (7)
Thoracic Vertebrae (12) — Spine
Lumbar Vertebrae (5)
Sacrum
Coccyx
Ischium
Tibia
Fibula

BACK

About Chakras

One of the reasons yoga is so good for the body, mind, and soul is because it works with various chakras in the body. The seven major chakras, according to yoga philosophy, receive, process, and distribute energy, affecting primarily the nervous and endocrine systems. The endocrine system controls the flow of hormones that determine growth rate, sexual development, and numerous physiological activities, and if it's operating well, you'll feel better all over. A well-toned nervous system informs you when to relax and when to take action.

When the flow of energy is balanced through the chakras, the mind-body system operates more positively. Yoga asanas or postures help balance the chakras. The result is a feeling of lightness, bliss, health, and a connection between ourselves and our environment.

Chakras also have connections to colors, sounds, emotions, glands, organs, elements, stages of development, and even certain rights of entitlement.

The first chakra, the *muladhara* or base chakra, is located at the base of the spine. It's associated with survival: being fed, sheltered, loved, cared for, and secure. Smell is the primary sense associated with *muladhara;* its color is red; its element is earth; and its right is to have.

The second chakra, called *svadhisthana,* is located in the lower abdomen. It's associated with our emotions and sexuality. Taste is the primary sense associated with *svadhisthana;* its color is orange; its element is water; and its right is to feel.

The third chakra, called *manipura,* is located in the solar plexus. This "abdominal brain" is the home of personal power, integrity, and gut feelings. When children are supported and nurtured in positive ways, their self-esteem is reinforced along with a sense of "I can do it!" Power is the primary quality associated with *manipura;* its color is yellow; its element is fire; and its right is to act.

The fourth chakra, called *anahata,* is located in the chest. The heart chakra is identified with love, compassion, and forgiveness. Dynamic breathing, positive relationships, and a love of self help maintain a healthy heart, boost the immune system, and encourage healing. Touch is the primary sense associated with *anahata;* its color is green; its element is air; and its right is to love.

The fifth chakra, called *vishuddha,* is located in the throat. The throat chakra is associated with expression, communication and creativity. It is associated with the thyroid, which regulates the child's growth and development. Hearing is the primary sense associated with *vishuddha;* its color is blue; its element is sound; and its right is to speak.

The sixth chakra, called *ajna,* is located between the eyebrows. Associated with clairvoyance, intuition, and imagination, the *ajna* chakra guides our dreams, our insights, our view of the world, and our place in it. It is associated with the pineal gland, which influences both the endocrine and central nervous systems. When the energy in this chakra flows freely, headaches and eye problems can be avoided. Sight is the primary sense of *ajna;* its color is indigo; its element is light; and its right is to see.

The seventh chakra, called *sahashara,* is located at the crown of the head. It is associated with knowledge and understanding. Our connection to our higher self—whether it be a higher state of being, nature, spirit, or god—flows through this chakra. The physical meets the spiritual at this chakra. Here lies the seat of the pituitary or master gland, which oversees all of the body's functions and systems. Pure being and knowing is the primary sense of *sahashara;* its color is violet; its element is thought; and its right is to know.

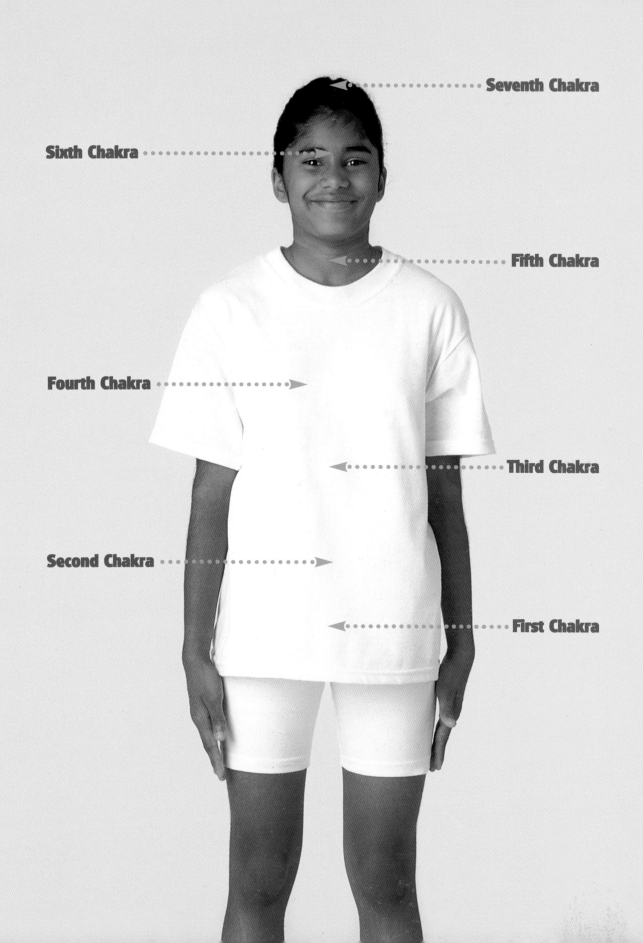

Seventh Chakra

Sixth Chakra

Fifth Chakra

Fourth Chakra

Third Chakra

Second Chakra

First Chakra

Visualization: A Magical Cloud Carpet Ride

Visualizations can help relax your child, especially during *savasana,* or Corpse pose. The effect is a lot like listening to a bedtime story. When you read this visualization, keep the lights and your voice low. Use soft, expressive tones. Play gentle and relaxing music in the background to set the mood. You can cover your child with a light blanket if the room is chilly and use an eye pillow if she likes it.

You may want to vary the script on occasion. Just substitute different places to visit, or invite your child to choose other countries and even planets to travel to.

Lie in *savasana.* Close your eyes and relax. Feel your body getting lighter and lighter as your breath fills you like a balloon and then gently escapes. Imagine your body so light and so relaxed that you just rise off the floor. Underneath you floats a beautiful, puffy, very comfortable cloud carpet. Just sink into your floating bed. It's a magical cloud carpet, and it will take you wherever you want to go.

Right alongside you—and you don't have to touch it now, just know that it's there and you can use it in your mind—is a little control panel or joystick, and you can take the cloud carpet up, down, or sideways, fast or slow, whatever you want to do, wherever you want to go.

As you continue to rise, feel the roof of the room open, and take your magical cloud carpet up to float through the sky. You will feel lighter and lighter as you move higher and higher into the sky. Birds fly all around you, and you can feel their wings flapping and other children laughing. You drift with the birds and the clouds in the sky. Remember that you have your own controls; any time you want to take your magical cloud carpet down, you can.

Feel yourself flying over rivers, deserts, farms, mountains, forests, beautiful fields filled with wildflowers—can you smell them? Smile or send kisses to all of the animals and trees.

You think you smell cotton candy, elephant ears, and other treats. You see lights and notice there is a carnival below you. Take your magical cloud carpet down to check it out. Park your carpet. Take a ride on the Ferris wheel or the carousel, drive some bumper cars, and hear some music. Play a few games. Get back on your carpet and fly up and away again. You can take your magical cloud carpet down into a cave and sit quietly with the bears inside, or float on a river, or go wherever you want to go.

You can visit your grandma or a friend in a faraway place. Perhaps you want to take a trip to outer space and see another planet or galaxy. In the next few minutes you have all the time you need to go where your heart desires.

You notice that it's beginning to get dark, and you wouldn't want your parents to worry about you, so you decide to head home. Turn your magical cloud carpet around and head back as you watch the sun set over the horizon. The stars begin to twinkle. You are so close to them that you can reach out and touch them. The moon warms and lights up your body with a golden glow.

(after a few minutes of silence)

You are now flying back into your town. You see your street and recognize your house: it's the

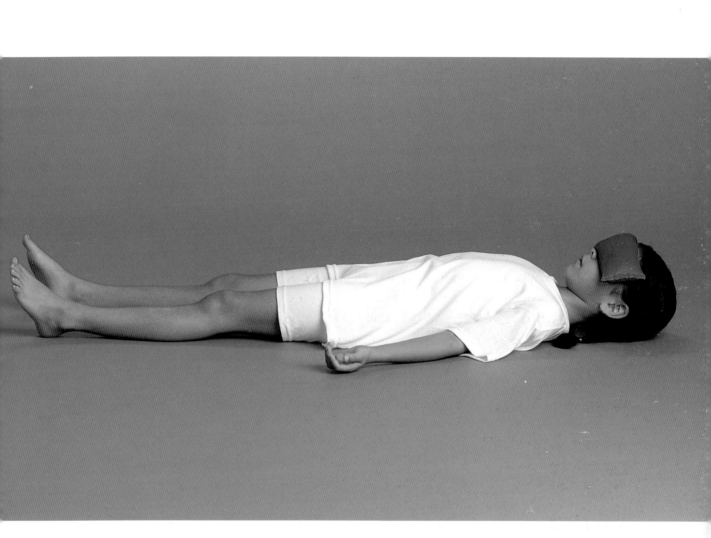

one with the open roof. You lower yourself gently into your room and back down to the floor. The roof closes quietly. You make a yawning sound, "Ahhhhh," as your arms stretch above your head and your legs and toes lengthen. Roll onto your side as you curl up and smile to yourself. Rest for a few moments in this position. Keep your eyes closed. When you're ready, bring your hands to the floor and press yourself up to sitting.

The Sound of Om

Sit cross-legged or "pretzel" your legs as you breathe in and out. Form your lips into the letter O. As you breathe out, say the letter O. Do this quietly three times: "O, O, O." Bring your lips together and think of your favorite food. Try curling your tongue upward and putting the tip of your tongue behind your teeth or on the roof of your mouth as you think about strawberries, pizza, spaghetti, or ice cream—whatever you find scrumptious—and go "Mmm." Make the mmm sound three times. Put those two sounds together (the O and the mmm) and sing the sound, "Ommmm." Do this three times. Feel the Om dance throughout your body and throat, bringing a sense of happiness and peace. ●

YogaKids® with Special Needs

The healing and learning powers of yoga can have wonderful effects on children with special needs. Whether children have learning disabilities, nervous conditions, physical handicaps, or even illnesses such as cancer, their reaction to YogaKids® is almost always positive.

Often, these children have spent a lot of time in doctors' and therapists' offices, so I want our time together to be fun; a respite from "work." The YogaKids way is to initiate and guide a process that is innately therapeutic without the tension and expectation. Even if the poses cannot be attained through children's own efforts, their bodies can be guided and supported in the yoga movements. Either way, they're still creating pathways and activating neurons in the brain.

Autism

For a child with autism the key is to create a strong bond. Yoga improves feelings of connection, enhances motor and communication skills, and can do wonders for a child's self-esteem. Don't feel that you have to dive right into doing the poses; play music or dance a little. Once your child is at ease, you can continue introducing different poses. Pattern, repetition, and trust are the key elements here.

Start slow. Work on base poses and breathing methods from the Peace & Quiet group. Once your child is comfortable with the concept of yoga, and the unfamiliar poses become familiar, gradually add more poses. Because visual stimulation and creating connections is important to autistic children, try this: Line up stuffed animals or pictures of animals at the front of the room. Follow the line of animals, doing the poses that relate to each one. The connection between the animal and the pose creates an effective pattern for your child.

For lower-functioning children, baskets of animal toys work better. Let your child choose an animal from the basket, and then do the pose that corresponds with the animal. Use the elements or pose groups in this book to create sequences to follow. Together, you can design a Transformer series of your own to reinforce patterns and rhythm.

Attention Deficit Disorder and Attention Deficit Hyperactivity Disorder

Children with ADD and ADHD have one primary difficulty—focus. Since focus is at the very core of yoga, it might seem nearly impossible to convince your attention-deficit child to hold still in a pose for more than a moment, but you'll find the act of doing yoga is often enough to hold her attention.

This might come as a surprise, but the best thing for attention-deficit children is *regular practice*. At least two to three times a week is optimal: the kids in our classes generally have about an hour, and practice with their parents as well. The key is to mix it up. Try making cards with photos of your child doing poses or with drawings of the poses (a tree, a dog, and so on) and number the groups of cards. Your child can pick a different group of cards or poses for each session.

As far as which poses to use, you'll probably want to avoid loud or fast poses because they're likely to overexcite an attention-deficit child. However, poses that require a lot of concentration and strength—like the Warrior series and the balance group, Feathers—will help your child focus. Lemon Toes is calming and works wonders. Eye pillows and breathing exercises will also relax your child. The combination of breathing methods with poses helps attention-deficit children develop greater body awareness, emotional balance, and concentration, increasing their capacity for schoolwork and creative play.

Cerebral Palsy

Because children with cerebral palsy are most affected in movement and posture, their muscles are often extremely tight. Holding a pose or a gentle stretch in yoga actually relaxes muscles, reduces high muscle tone, and exercises the areas of low muscle tone. Because kids with cerebral palsy often have breathing problems, focus on breathing and strengthening stomach muscles, as well.

The primary benefit of yoga for these kids, though, is the stretching and realignment of the spine. Poses like Twist and Blow, Sit and Twist, and many in the Strength & Courage and Shape & Form categories exercise the spine in many ways, lengthening the space between vertebrae and relaxing pressure on nerves throughout the body. This offers the dual benefit of releasing muscular tension and enhancing overall nerve function, which gives your child more movement, coordination, and flexibility.

One of our CYKFs says that a method she calls "Log Rolling" does wonders for her kids with CP. Get a bolster or rolled-up blanket, and have your child lie back on it with her arms resting out to the side. Then gently, slowly, rock the log back and forth. Kids find it funny and relaxing. No child has ever disliked this pose, and it's a chance to energize the spine and try to open the front of a body that has a tendency to stay hunched.

Down's Syndrome

Because children with Down's syndrome generally have shorter limbs and delayed cognitive development, YogaKids works on both physical and mental abilities. As with any developmental disability, yogic breathing exercises can always improve the central nervous system and help develop body awareness, concentration, and memory. Use the Peace & Quiet group, as well as Brain Balance poses. In addition, Four-Legged Friends and Strength & Courage poses stabilize joints, bolster integrity in the connective tissue, and build muscle strength and tone.

Try using the walls and floor as a "backbone" of support in poses like L Is for Left, Tree, and Mountain. The more "buttressed" the ligaments of the spine, neck, and head, the greater the benefits.

Affirmations

An affirmation is a positive statement about oneself. It can be broad or very specific. In YogaKids® we like to add affirmations to our poses in order to connect the verbal and physical expressions of our feelings. It's a way of putting into words the qualities our pose can inspire in us. Below are some affirmations we use with the poses in this book (others are printed with the pose instructions). Use this list as a beginning: Once they get the idea, children like to create their own affirmations.

(from Handstands, pages 98–99)
I am confident.
I am brave.
I can do anything.

(from Reach for the Sun, pages 86–87)
I can hold my power.
The sun shines upon me. The sun shines within me.
When I feel insecure, I reach for the sun.
When I feel afraid, I turn on the light inside of me.

(from Take 5, page 26)
When I get upset, I take five.
When I get frustrated, I take five.
Before a test, I take five to quiet my brain
 and focus my mind.

(from Peace Breath, page 25)
I am peace.
I am kind.
I help others.
Peace begins within me.

(from Wheel, page 91)
I am flexible.
My heart is open.
My spine is strong.
My brain is alert.

(from Warrior Series, pages 54–55)
I am strong.
I am powerful.
I can live my heart's desire. YES!!

Song Lyrics

Here are lyrics to some of the songs suggested in the poses. Make this list a starting point for your child's own collection of favorite songs. The music chart (page 114) can lead to you to new songs to add to your collection.

(from Om a Little Teapot Triangle, page 88)
Om a Little Teapot
Om a little teapot, short and stout.
Here is my handle.
Here is my spout.
When I get all steamed up, I reach out.
Then tip me over and pour me up.

(from Rocking Horse page 90)
The Rocking Horse Song
Oh, rocking horse,
Front to back
Front to back
Rocking horse stays on track.

(Music and lyrics by Joel Frankel, 1993, from the audio *Don't Sit on a Cactus.*)

(from Row Your Boat, page 78)
Row, Row, Row Your Boat
Row, row, row your boat
Gently down the stream.
Merrily, merrily, merrily, merrily,
Life is but a dream.

(from Bug-Pickin' Chimp, page 71)
Sing to the melody of "Five Little Monkeys."

Bug pickin' chimps went swinging through the trees
They laughed and sang and breathed "he-he."
Cleaned their fur till their coats were nit-free
Then shared big bananas for all to see.

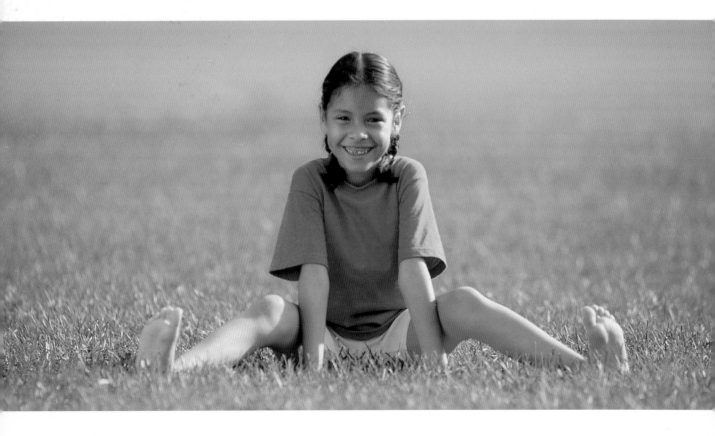

A YogaKids® class generally ends with the Namaste song: You can do the same at home. Either play the YogaKids tape or CD and sing along with the words listed below or sing it a capella (without accompaniment). Instructions for movements that go along with the words are written under each of the lyric lines.

Namaste Song

I am you and you are me
[point or gesture with your hand toward yourself and then to someone else]

I am part of all I see
[raise your hands above your head, and wiggle your fingers as you turn around in a circle]

Namaste, Namaste, Namaste, Namaste
[put your hands together at your heart and bow to another person each time you say "Namaste"]

I am the light and the light is me
[point or gesture toward yourself and then to the sun; point or gesture toward the sun and then to yourself]

Namaste, Namaste, Namaste, Namaste
[put your hands together at your heart and bow to another person each time you say "Namaste"]

I shine bright with all I see
[Move your Namaste hands upward like you do in Volcano. Separate them, arc your arms outward through the air, and return them to your heart in the Namaste position]

The light in me sees the light in you
[Gently touch your hand to your heart, palm down, and extend your arm out to point or gesture toward another person with an open hand]

Bow to me, I'll bow to you
[place your hands together at your heart and bow to that person]

The light in me sees the light in you
[this time choose a different person to point or gesture toward and bow]

Bow to me, I'll bow to you
[place your hands together at your heart and bow toward that person]

Namaste, Namaste, Namaste, Namaste
[repeat]

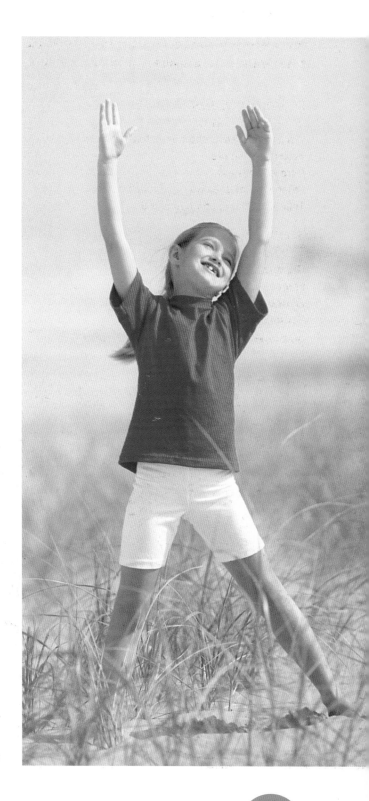

Musical Musings

Although many people associate yoga with silence—and that's a big part of it—music can be valuable too. As a matter of fact, in the YogaKids® program, it's integral. Playing our own instruments, singing nursery rhymes, hissing like snakes, chanting our names, and pounding our chests Tarzan-style are just a few musical interludes that are part of our program.

We blend our own sounds with recorded music. No matter what music we use, or when or how we use it, music is a vital part of how children learn and a vital aspect of this program. We like to include all types of music—energizing as well as calming, catchy as well as unfamiliar. Music sets appropriate moods for the children, so it's a great tool. (I find it's essential for children with autism.)

Music is a powerful hook to memory, activates neural pathways, and triggers a host of connections in the brain. Not only will using a variety of familiar and unfamiliar tunes encourage your child's love of yoga, but it will also lay the groundwork for a lifetime of music appreciation!

Here are four pages of examples of how we use music. Experiment; you'll find what works for you and your child.

POSE	SONG	ALBUM	COMPOSER/ARTIST
Lizard	"Iguana"	*Animal Alphabet*	David S. Polansky
Moo and Meow	"The Cheshire Cat" and "Paw by Paw"	*Wander Down Beyond the Rainbow*	Mim Eichmann and Doug Lofstrom
	"Making Moosic"	*Making Moosic*	Anna Moo
Dromedary Delight	"Camels"	*Animal Alphabet*	David S. Polansky
Down Diggety Doggy Down	"Dog Rules"	*In My Hometown*	Tom Chapin
	"Who Let the Dogs Out"	*Who Let the Dogs Out*	Baha Men
ABC poses	"There Is Sound for Every Letter of the Alphabet"	*Share It!*	Rosenshontz
	"A—You're Adorable"	*Singin' in the Bathtub*	John Lithgow
S Is for Snake/ Snake Charmer	"Boa Constrictor" (poem by Shel Silverstein)	*Five Little Monkeys*	Dennis Buck
R Is for Roar	"Pet Sounds"	*Share It!*	Rosenshontz
L Is for Left	"La La La"	*Sesame Street Sing the Alphabet*	

POSE	SONG	ALBUM	COMPOSER/ARTIST
Brain Balance poses	"The Balancing Act"	*Kids in Motion*	Kevin Quinn
Twist and Blow	"Twist and Shout"	*Please Please Me*	The Beatles
Eagle	"Eagle's Journey"	*Tribal Winds*	
Feathers poses	"Bird Bath Buddies"	*Wander Down Beyond the Rainbow*	Mim Eichmann and Doug Lofstrom
	"Birdland"	*Extensions*	The Manhattan Transfer
Stork	"Lullaby of Birdland"	*Snoopy's Jazz Classiks on Toys*	
Flamingo	"Tweet Tweet"	*Making Moosic*	Anna Moo
360-Degree Owl	"The Owl"	*Improvise with Eric Nagler*	Eric Nagler
Crow	"The Thieving Magpie"		Rossini
Strength & Courage poses	"Ain't No Mountain High Enough"	*The Very Best of Marvin Gaye*	Marvin Gaye
Mountain	"The World's Greatest"	*Ali: Original Soundtrack*	R Kelly
Volcano	"Volcano"	*The Parakeet Album*	W. O. Smith Music School Singers
	"Volcano"	*Songs of Jimmy Buffett*	Jimmy Buffet
Warrior Series	"The Young Old Warrior"	*Emergence*	Carlos Nakai
Tree	"Paint with All the Colors of the Wind" (instrumental)	*Heigh Ho! Mozart*	Donald Fraser, arranger
Edible poses	"Tummy Tango"	*Kids in Motion*	
Peanut Butter & Jelly	"My Body Machine"	*My Body Machine*	Janeen Brady
Completion poses	"Namaste"	*Music from YogaKids®*	Chris Bennett and Marsha Wenig
Magical Cloud Carpet Ride	"To Touch the Sky"	*Chrysalis*	2002

POSE	SONG	ALBUM	COMPOSER/ARTIST
Row Your Boat	"Sailing to the Sea"	*Mother Earth*	Tom Chapin
	"Row, Row, Row Your Boat"	*Row Row Row Your Boat*	Various artists
Talking Turtle	"Tortoises"	*Carnival of the Animals*	Camille Saint-Saëns
Spouting Dolphin	"The Trout"	*Children's Favourites*	Liszt (on a theme by Schubert)/ Julius Katchen
Bubble Fish	"Aquarium"	*Carnival of the Animals*	Camille Saint-Saëns
Ankle-Heel-Toe Walking	"New Way to Walk"	*Hot Hot Hot Dance Songs*	Sesame Street
Bug-Pickin' Chimp		*Sounds of the Tropical Rain Forest*	Gentle Persuasion
	"Zoo Blues"	*Brasil*	The Manhattan Transfer
Roller Coaster	"Me and Bobby McGee"	*Pearl*	Janis Joplin
Shake Like Jelly	"Shake Your Bootie Wootie"	*Making Moosic*	Anna Moo
		Deep Forest	Deep Forest
Untying the Knots	"Thinkin' About Your Body"	*Spontaneous Inventions*	Bobby McFerrin
Ragoll Ann and Ragdoll Andy	"Morning's Rag"	*Guitar Lullaby*	Ricardo Cobo
Peace & Quiet poses	"Along the Path"	*Wander Down Beyond the Rainbow*	Mimi Eichmann and Doug Lofstrom
Hot Air Balloon	"Magic Kite"	*Snoopy's Jazz Classiks* Classiks on Toys	
Child's Pose		*Music to Be Born By*	Micky Hart
Swim Ducky Swim	"The Swan"	*The Carnival of Animals*	Camille Saint-Saëns
Take 5	"Take Five"	*Time Out*	Dave Brubeck Quartet

POSE	SONG	ALBUM	COMPOSER/ARTIST
Butterfly	"Monarch Butterfly"	Songs about Insects, Bugs, and Squiggly Things	Kimbo
Shape & Form poses		Journey in Satchidananda	Alice Coltrane
Rocking Horse	"Rocking Horse"	Don't Sit on a Cactus	Joel Frankel
Connecting poses	"Circle of Life"	Lion King: Original Motion Picture Soundtrack	Elton John and Tim Rice
Partner Twists		Beyond Words	Bobby McFerrin
Electric Circle	"In Harmony"	Sesame Street: In Harmony	Sesame Street
Pattern & Rhythm	"J'Aime Percussion"	Elmo and the Orchestra	Charles Brissette and Edvard Mitchell
	"The Wheel of the Water"	Mother Earth	Tom Chapin
Transformers	"Footprints"	Footprints	Jai Uttal
Reach for the Sun	"Reach for the Sun"	Music from YogaKids®	Chris Bennett and Marsha Wenig
Senses poses		A Love Supreme	John Coltrane
Eyes Around the Clock	"Rock Around the Clock"	Rock Around the Clock	Bill Haley and His Comets
Pedal Laughing	"Everybody Has a Laughing Place"	The Music of Disney— A Legacy in Song	Ray Gilbert and Alli Wrobel
Tarzan's Thymus Tap	"Tarzan"	Tarzan: An Original Walt Disney Record	Mark Mancina and Phil Collins
Upside Down poses		Kind of Blue	Miles Davis
Birthday Candle Series	"Happy Birthday"	Great Big Fun for the Very Little One	Tom Chapin
Lemon Toes	"Popsicle Toes"	The Best of Michael Franks: A Backward Glance	Michael Franks

Music for Lemon Toes or as nice background to a session

Deva Premal, Embrace

Miles Davis, Kind of Blue

Rasa, Devotion

Libera, Libera

Secret Garden, Songs from a Secret Garden

Marina Ray, Blissful Journey

Reading Comes Alive with Yoga

There are few better ways to get children to love books than to let them pretend to be in one; in a nutshell, that's what this element does. Not only is your child reading, but you're also reading together, absorbing the story, doing yoga poses, and exercising your body and brain muscles all at once. It's a great way to add the visual, language and brain balance elements, and to integrate your yoga sessions with reading enrichment.

You can use this element in more than one way: Read the book together and then go back and choose poses from this book that are relevant to the story. Or just jump right in; reading, acting out the story, trying a related pose, or connecting to other elements by drawing, painting, or counting.

You won't just read the book from start to finish: This is interactive reading, doing poses that coincide with the story, so don't worry if you don't make it all the way through the book in one session. If you're using a book about trees, such as Shel Silverstein's *The Giving Tree* or Lynn Cherry's *The Great Kapok Tree,* go outside and sit under a tree while reading it. And then do the Tree Pose, and all the other applicable poses in the story. If you select a book about anatomy, perhaps *Dem Bones* by Bob Barner or *Your Insides* by Joanna Cole, touch and say those parts, draw them, and talk about what they do. Practice poses that use them.

Although most Reading Comes Alive selections are movement-oriented, there are some that spotlight other important elements, such as Sarah Perry's *If, The Loveables in the the Kingdom of Self Esteem* by Diane Loomis, or two books by Nancy Carlson, *I Like Me* and *ABC I Like Me.* Other favorites in this category are *How Are you Peeling?* by Joost Elfers, *Today I Feel Silly* by Jamie Lee Curtis and Laura Cornell, *My Many Colored Days* by Dr. Seuss, and *Hey Little Ant* by Hannah and Phillip Hoose. During class, we sometimes just read the books with only a handful of movements, spending most of our time on activities from the Laughing Language, Quiet Quests, Affirmations or Visual Vignette elements.

The following pages contain more than 80 books for you to choose from. About half of them are linked to specific poses from this book, providing an appropriate Reading Comes Alive element for any sequence. The rest of the list is more general—use these titles to enhance any theme or element in your session.

POSE	TITLE	AUTHOR/ILLUS.	SUMMARY
Lizard	*Lizard in the Sun*	Joanne Ryder; illustrated by Michael Rothman	Become a lizard for a day.
Moo and Meow, Feathers poses, Tree	*Feathers for Lunch*	Lois Ehlert	Prowling cat adventure.
Moo and Meow, Down Diggety Doggy Down, Lemon Toes	*Cock A Doodle Moo*	Bernard Most	Sick rooster enlists cow to wake up the farm.
Dromedary Delight, Bunny Breath, S Is for Snake/Snake Charmer, Talking Turtle, Tree, 360-Degree Owl, Rocking Horse	*Benjamin Dilley's Thirsty Camel*	Jolly Roger Bradfield	Dreamer's wonderful imagination.

POSE	TITLE	AUTHOR/ILLUS.	SUMMARY
Down Diggety Doggy Down, Moo and Meow, Swim Ducky Swim	*Bark, George*	Jules Feiffer	Mom wants George to bark, but he keeps making other animal noises.
ABC poses, Bug-Pickin' Chimp, Swim Ducky Swim, Flamingo, Rocking Horse, Talking Turtle	*"A" is for ---? A Photographer's Alphabet/Animals*	Henry Horenstein	Dazzling photographic wild animal puzzle.
S Is for Snake/Snake Charmer, Tree, Bubble Fish, Feathers poses, Lemon Toes	*Verdi*	Jannell Cannon	Python doesn't want to grow old and boring.
Tree, Take 5	*The Lion Who Had Asthma*	Jonathan London; illustrated by Nadine Bernard Westcott	Boy with asthma uses relaxation and imagination.
Twist and Blow, any standing poses with twisting	*The Straight Line Wonder*	Mem Fox; illustrated by Marc Rosenthal	Independent-spirited line wants to twirl and twist.
Eagle, Bubble Fish, Row Your Boat, Warrior Series, Spouting Dolphin	*Eagle Boy*	Richard Lee Vaughn; illustrated by Lee Christiansen	Pacific Northwest Indians and eagles come to live in harmony.
Bow and Arrow, Feathers poses	*Feathers and Fools*	Mem Fox; illustrated by Nicholas Wilton	Escalation of arms/war, and return of peace.
Feathers poses, S Is for Snake/Snake Charmer, Lizard, Talking Turtle, Bubble Fish, Butterfly	*Chickens Aren't the Only Ones*	Ruth Heller	Oviparous egg layers— fascinating illustrations.
360-Degree Owl, Tree, Butterfly, Moo and Meow, Bunny Breath, S Is for Snake/Snake Charmer, Polar Bear	*The Owl who Became the Moon*	Jonathan London; illustrated by Ted Rand	Boy's magical journey through moonlit snowy night.
Flamingo	*For Pete's Sake*	Ellen Stoll Walsh	Pete, an alligator, worries about how he's different.
Volcano, Take 5, Peace Breath	*Sometimes I'm a Bombaloo*	Rachel Vail; illustrated by Yumi Heo	Importance of calming down after angy outbursts.
Tree, Swinging Pretzel	*The Giving Tree*	Shel Silverstein	Sustaining gifts of tree to child.
Polar Bear, any posture that emphasizes top, bottom, or middle	*Tops and Bottoms*	Janet Stevens	Trickster rabbit beats hardship by his wits.

POSE	TITLE	AUTHOR/ILLUS.	SUMMARY
Lemon Toes, visualizations	*The Next Place*	Warren Hanson	Vision of heavenly peace.
Lemon Toes, Moo and Meow, Swim Ducky Swim, Rocking Horse, Child's Pose	*Going to Sleep on the Farm*	Wendy Cheyette Lewison; illustrated by Juan Wijngaard	Boy asks his father how farm animals prepare for sleep.
Wet poses, Talking Turtle	*Fireflies, Fireflies, Light My Way*	Jonathan London; illustrated by Linda Messier	Inspired by a Mesaqakioe lullaby of magical pond.
Row Your Boat, Wet poses	*Bobby Otter and the Blue Boat*	Margaret Burdick	Otter desperately wants to trade badger for boat.
Talking Turtle, Tree, Feathers poses, Bubble Fish, Mountain, Polar Bear, Butterfly	*Old Turtle*	Douglas Wood; illustrated by Cheng-Khee Chee	Fable that probes the nature of interconnections.
Polar Bear, Flamingo, S Is for Snake/Snake Charmer	*Polar Bear, Polar Bear, What do You Hear?*	Bill Martin Jr.; illustrated by Eric Carle	Children imitate zoo animal sounds.
Bubble Fish	*Rainbow Fish*	Marcus Pfister and J. Alison James	Cautionary tale about vanity and friendship.
Moving & Grooving poses	*From Head to Toe*	Eric Carle	Stomp, thump, and bend with playful characters.
Ankle-Heel-Toe Walking, Bunny Breath, Moo and Meow, Dromedary Delight, Rocking Horse	*What Neat Feet*	Hana Machotka	Specialization of the feet that connect us to earth.
Peace & Quiet poses, Tree, Wet poses, Feathers poses	*Grandad's Prayers of the Earth*	Wood, Douglas; illustrated by P. J. Lynch	Trees, rocks, and birds pray and reach for heaven.
Hot Air Balloon, Bug-Pickin' Chimp, Mountain	*Curious George and the Hot Air Balloon*	Margret Rey; illustrated by Vipah Interactive	George takes a hot air balloon and saves a worker.
Swim Ducky Swim, S Is for Snake (props on abdomen)	*Little White Duck*	Walt Whippo (lyrics); illustrated by Joan Paley (music by Bernard Zaritzky)	Mouse narrates beloved song.
Dragon Breath, S Is for Snake, Rocking Horse	*"The Grateful Snake" in Crocodile, Crocodile*	Barbara Baumgartner; illustrated by Judith Moffatt	Magical dragon helps generous boy.
Take 5, Tree, Row Your Boat, Feathers poses, Rocking Horse, Bubble Fish, Mountain, Polar Bear	*A Quiet Place*	Douglas Wood; illustrated by Dan Andreason	Discover the very best quiet place of all—inside.

POSE	TITLE	AUTHOR/ILLUS.	SUMMARY
Butterfly	*Waiting for Wings*	Lois Ehlert	Arresting artwork showing butterfly.
Shape & Form poses, Om a Little Teapot	*Color Zoo*	Lois Ehlert	Making an art zoo, using shapes and colors.
Rocking Horse	*Rocking Horse Angel*	Mercer Mayer	Enchanted rocking horse guides feverish boy "home."
Connecting poses, Swinging Pretzel, Tree, 360-Degree Owl	*The Kissing Hand*	Audrey Penn; illustrated by Ruth E. Harper and Nancy M. Leak	Gentle, reassuring way to say, "You are loved."
Transformers	*Babar's Yoga for Elephants*	Laurent De Brunhoff	Babar demonstrates daily hatha yoga routine.
Senses poses	*The Other Way to Listen*	Byrd Baylord; illustrated by Peter Parnall	Attuning to nature's subtle songs.
Upside down poses, Tree, Moo and Meow, Lizard, Bug-Pickin' Chimp, Feathers poses, Talking Turtle	*Slowly, Slowly, Slowly, Said the Sloth*	Eric Carle	A sloth hangs upside down while animals speed by.
Handstands (any inversion)	*Reflections*	Ann Jonas	Art book with playful upside-down view on each page.
Birthday Candle Series, Swinging Pretzel, Bubble Fish, Reach for the Sun	*Birthdays! Celebrating Life Around the World*	Eve B. Feldman; illustrated by Paintbrush Diplomacy	Ways of celebrating around the world.
Reach for the Sun, Child's Pose, Ragdoll Ann and Ragdoll Andy, Lemon Toes	*Claude and the Sun*	Matt Novak	Claude's best friend is the sun. They grow flowers, play, and sleep together.
Eyes Around the Clock, Moo and Meow, Lizard, Child's Pose	*Telling Time with Big Mama Cat*	Dan Harper; illustrated by Barry and Cara Moser	Cat recounts grueling schedule of napping, stretching, and prewashing dishes to movable clock.
Pedal Laughing, Polar Bear	Don't Make Me Laugh	James Stevenson	Preschool book sure to make the young giggle.
Om a Little Teapot, Wheel, and any pose that emphasizes shapes	*A Triangle for Adaora: An African Book of Shapes*	Ifeoma Onyefulu	Cousin goes through village in search of a triangle for Adaora.

Favorite Books of YogaKids®

ABC I Like Me, Nancy Carlson

All I See Is Part of Me, Chara M. Curtis; illustrated by Cynthia Aldrich

Audrey and Barbara, Janet Lawson

Badger's Parting Gift, Susan Varley

The Circle of Days, Reeve Lindberg; illustrated by Cathie Felstead

Click Clack Moo: Cows That Type, Doreen Cronin; illustrated by Betsy Lewin

Color Farm, Lois Ehlert

Daddy, Could I Have an Elephant, Jake Wolf; illustrated by Marylin Hafner

Each Living Thing, Joanne Ryder

Hey Little Ant, Hannah and Phillip Hoose

How Are You Peeling?, Joost Elfers

Hush! A Thai Lullaby, Minfong Ho; illustrated by Holly Meade

The Icky Sticky Frog, Dawn Bentley

If, Sarah Perry

I Look Like a Tiger, Sheila Hamanaka

I'm a Tiger, Too, Marie-Louise Fitzpatrick

Is This a House for Hermit Crab?, Megan McDonald

The Loveables in the Kingdom of Self-Esteem, Diane Loomans

Mama, Do You Love Me?, Barbara Joosse

The Mixed Up Chameleon, Eric Carle

My Many Colored Days, Dr. Seuss

On the Day You Were Born, Debra Frasier

Owl Moon, Jane Yolen; illustrated by John Schoenherr

Parts!, Tedd Arnold

Peter and the Pigeons, Charlotte Zolotow; illustrated by Martine Gourbault

Return of the Shadows, Norma Farber; illustrated by Andrea Baruffi

The Runaway Bunny, Margaret Wise Brown

Sun Song, Jean Marzollo; illustrated by Laura Regan

There's an Alligator under My Bed, Mercer Mayer

Today I Feel Silly, Jamie Lee Curtis

When Will It Be Spring?, Catherine Walters

Where the Wild Things Are, Maurice Sendak

Children's Anatomy Books

A Book about Your Skeleton, Ruth Belov Gross

Brain Surgery for Beginners, Steve Parker and David West

Dem Bones, Bob Barner

How Your Body Works, Jo Ellen More

My Five Senses, Aliki Brandenberg

Outside and Inside You, Sandra Markle

The Skeleton Inside of You, Philip Balestrino

Your Insides, Joanna Cole

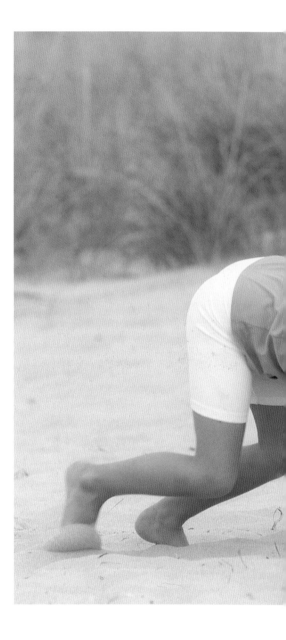

Branches of Your Brain

Imagine a tree, with branches reaching out to send and retrieve information: the roots of the tree are your brain, and the trunk is your spinal cord. The branches are the nerves in your body, picking up sensations and sending them back to your brain for processing.

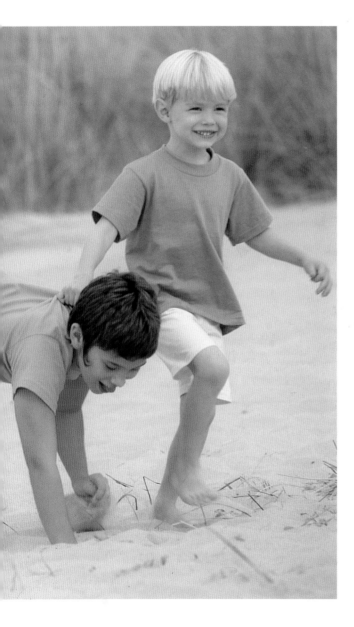

This "tree" made up of the brain, spinal cord, and nerves is called the central nervous system. It's an amazing system, and yoga can help you become more in tune with it. Not only will you understand your body's signals better, but you'll also improve the efficiency and clarity of the system.

The brain is made up of three parts, all of which control different functions in your body. The first one, located in the brain stem just above the back of your neck, is often called the base or "reptilian" brain. It controls the most basic functions like breathing, heartbeat, and instinctual responses to danger or safety. The central part of our brain is referred to as the limbic system, or mammalian brain. Its realm is emotions, sexuality, and memory. The top layer of our brain, the neocortex—literally, "new bark"—is what makes us uniquely human. The neocortex is further divided into two hemispheres, and each hemisphere emphasizes a different set of strengths. The corpus callosum links the two halves; it's like a communication highway between left and right brains. Brain Balance poses and elements help your child "exercise" his corpus callosum. Because he's using both sides of his brain, the communication between halves is more active.

The left side of the brain emphasizes language, logic, numbers, mathematics, sequence, and words: the academic aspects of learning. The right side emphasizes rhyme, rhythm, music, pictures, imagination, and patterns: the creative aspects of learning. Both halves are equally essential, and the YogaKids® whole-child approach strives to keep them in balance.

Each area of the brain has its own specialty: seeing, hearing, touching, moving, and so on. When we practice yoga—and especially when we use the YogaKids elements—we create a fertile atmosphere for learning. Every time we practice our asanas and use the elements of YogaKids, we create new "branches" for neurotransmitters, and new ways to learn.

The YogaKids® Classroom Experience

In a YogaKids class, a Certified YogaKids Facilitator (CYKF) not only instructs the children but also guides them and helps to give full play to their yoga.

The connection between the facilitator and the children enables a genuine growth of mutual health, humanity, love, and understanding of their bodies and minds. We don't give tests in YogaKids classes, but over time we can see the children's improvement. The curriculum and class environment naturally support and reinforce children's innate ability to learn and succeed. Each child develops a sense of achievement and confidence in her creativity and experience in every moment.

The class format integrates all of the YogaKids elements. It includes poses, movement, anatomy, breathing techniques, music, cooperative games, partner play, Reading Comes Alive, relaxation, and an art or language project. Classes are thematic: Night Animals, Gratitude, Friends, and Anatomy and Me are just a few examples of the hundreds of lesson plans shared within the CYKF network. Most important, facilitators and children are always learning from each other, and enjoying themselves, too.

To find a CYKF in your area or become one yourself, go to http://www.yogakids.com.

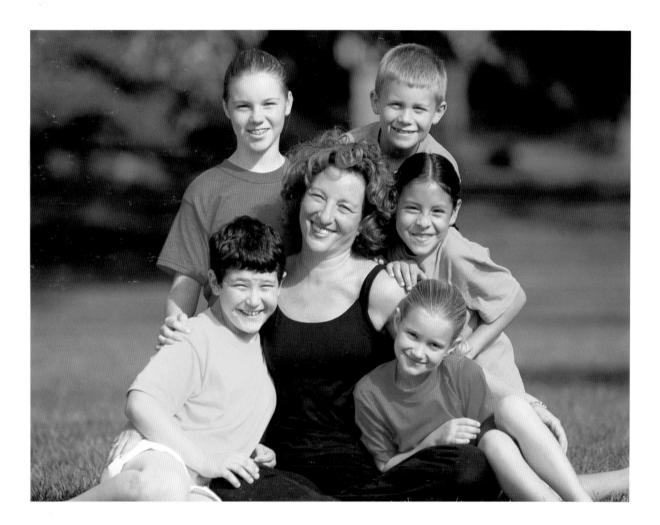

Books on Yoga, Children, and Teaching

The books listed below have informed and inspired me as I developed YogaKids®:

Brain-Based Learning, Eric Jensen. (Brain Store Inc., 2000)

Brain Gym (Teacher's Edition), Paul E. Dennison, and Gail E. Dennison. (Edu Kinesthetics, 1994)

Children's Atlas of the Human Body: Actual Size Bones, Muscles, and Organ in Full Color, Richard Walker. (Millbrook Publishers, 1994)

Children's Book of Yoga: Games & Exercises Mimic Plants & Animals & Objects, Thia Luby. (Clear Light Publishers, 1998)

A Child's Garden of Yoga, Baba Hari Dass.(Sri Rama Publishers, 1980)

Eight Ways of Knowing: Teaching for Multiple Intelligences, David Lazear. (SkyLight Professional Development, 1998)

Eight Ways of Teaching: The Artistry of Teaching with Multiple Intelligences, David Lazear. (SkyLight Professional Development, 1998)

Frames of The Mind: The Theory of Multiple Intelligences, Howard Gardner. (Basic Books, 1993)

Hatha Yoga: Developing the Body, Mind and Inner Self, Dee A. Birkel. (Eddie Bowers Publishing Company, 1996)

The Heart of Yoga: Developing a Personal Practice, T.K.V. Desikachar. (Inner Traditions Intl. Ltd, 1999)

Gray's Anatomy: A Fact Filled Coloring Book, Freddy Stark. (Running Press, 2001)

Learning with the Body in Mind, Eric Jensen. (Brain Store Inc., 2000)

The Learning Revolution: A Lifelong Learning Program for the World's Finest Computer Your Amazing Brain, Gordon Dryden and Jeannette Vos, Ed.D. (Jalmar Press, 1994)

Living Your Yoga: Finding The Spiritual in Everyday Life, Judith Lasater. (Rodmell Press, 2000)

Light on Yoga: Yoga Dipika, B.K.S. Iyengar. (Schocken Books, 1995)

Magical Child, Joseph Chilton Pearce. (Plume, 1992)

The Sivananda Companion to Yoga: A Complete Guide to the Physical Postures, Breathing Exercises, Diet, Relaxation, and Meditation Techniques of Yoga, Swami Vishnu-Devananda. (Fireside, 2000)

Smart Moves: Why Learning Is Not All in Your Head, Carla Hannaford, Ph.D. (Great Ocean Publishers, 1995)

The Sevenfold Journey: Reclaiming Mind, Body & Spirit Through the Chakras, Anodea Judith and Selene Vega. (Crossing Press, 1993)

Spinning Inward: Using Guided Imagery with Children for Learning, Creativity & Relaxation, Maureen Murdock. (Shambhala Publications, 1988)

Tribes: A New Way of Learning and Being Together, Jeanne Gibbs. (CenterSource Systems, LLC, 2001)

Yoga for Children, Mary Stewart and Kathy Phillips. (Fireside, 1993)

Yoga for Children, Swati and Rajiv Chanchani. (UBS Publishers' Distributors Ltd., 1995)

Yoga for The Special Child: A Therapeutic Approach for Infants and Children with Down Syndrome, Cerebral Palsy, and Learning Disabilities, Sonia Sumar. (Special Yoga Publishers, 1998)

Yoga: The Path to Holistic Health, B.K.S Iyengar. (DK Publishing, 2001)

Yoga: The Poetry of The Body, Rodney Yee. (St. Martin's Press, 2002)

Yoga: The Spirit and Practice of Moving into Stillness, Erich Schiffman. (Pocket Books, 1996)

Acknowledgments

I am so grateful to so many for supporting and nurturing YogaKids®:

Thanks to my "special agent" Joy Tutela for her beauty, patience, wisdom and guidance; Jody Handley for helping me find my voice on paper; publisher Leslie Stoker for her enthusiasm and commitment; editor Anne Kostick for her assistance, understanding, and knowledge throughout this whole process; designer Susi Oberhelman for building a wonderama of color, texture, and invitation; publicist Caroline Enright and the production and marketing teams at STC.

Thanks to photographer Susan Andrews and her discriminating eye, and to those who supported us in making these beautiful photographs: Lisa Baruch, Donte' Tatem, Sue Torres, Kim Waldron, and the helpful parents of our young models.

Namaste to all the magnificent YogaKids for the beauty, patience and smiles that grace these pages: Sylvia Agba; Jyoti Gopal Bock; Devon Carlson; Griffin Carlson; Catherine Ford; Shelby Ford; Taylor Henderson; Alexandra Jacobson; Tommy McIlwaine; Zahara Schooley; James Servillas; Marissa Taebel; Andrea Torres; Marina Vulinovic; Ava Vulinovic; and Kiva Wenig.

Thanks to all my teachers who shared their wisdom and creativity in a multitude of ways throughout my life. Thanks especially to my husband Don for being such a great yoga teacher as well as my partner in love and life.

To all the people who fostered the growth of YogaKids with their support, belief and experience over the years: Amy Baker; Jeane Bock; Susan Branch and the Michigan City Public Library; Ally and Russ Ben Ezzer; Chris Bennett; Judian Breitenbach; Sandy Carden; Patty Carroll; Crichfield Elementary School, especially Mona Tisch and Pam McIntyre; Arlene and Alexandra Rosenberg DaSilva; Karen Dupuis; Amy Kline Gage; Micheal Glicksohn; Alan Goldberg; Michael Greenwald; Gail Grossman; Gladys and Avron Grossman; Adrienne Hamilton and Chicago HeadStart; Indiana Dunes National Lakeshore; Katie Ingersoll; Jonny Kest; Jodi Komitor; Angel Gail Konz; La Lumiere School; Charyl and Tom McComas; Stephanie and Gordon Medlock; Albert Nilam Meyerer and Kripalu; The Montessori School of Michigan City; Cathleen Pascale; Aunt Evie Preston; Ed and Sharon Raab; Nancy and Pius Ruby; Laurie Schaeffer; Pam Smith; Shelli Stein; Victoria Strohmeyer; Sonia (Sivakami) Sumar. Marcia and Tim Taebel; Monica Veneziano; Dakota Wenig; Norman and Janice Wenig; and Kathy and Walt Zmuda.

To the dedicated personnel of YogaKids International, for taking care of all the details: Misha Binzen; Cheryl Olen; Colin Spitler; and Kim Waldron.

Special thanks to Catherine Crowell, CYKF, for her creativity and support in the compilation of the music and Reading Comes Alive lists for this book.

To Summer Kopfmann for sharing her experience with her YogaKids at The Therapy Place and "log rolling."

To Rick Resnick for inspiring the Polar Bear pose and to Ally Peer Ben Ezzer, CYKF for the Roller Coaster pose.

In gratitude to our growing family of CYKFs for sharing their love and wisdom with children around the world: Thank you for being the best.

Index

Page numbers in **boldface** indicate major discussion of the topic. Those in *italics* indicate illustrations.